Treatment of Refractory Renal Anemia

Bi-Cheng Liu
Editor

Bin Wang
Associate Editor

Treatment of Refractory Renal Anemia

Case Collection

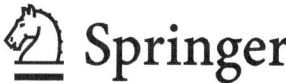
Springer

Editor
Bi-Cheng Liu
Institute of Nephrology
Zhongda Hospital, Southeast University
Nanjing, China

Associate Editor
Bin Wang
Department of Nephrology
Zhongda Hospital
Southeast University
Nanjing, China

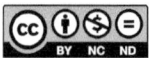

ISBN 978-981-97-7635-1   ISBN 978-981-97-7636-8   (eBook)
https://doi.org/10.1007/978-981-97-7636-8

This work was supported by Shanghai JiaYiHui Information Technology Co.

This Springer imprint is published by the registered company Springer Nature Singapore Pte Ltd.
The registered company address is: 152 Beach Road, #21-01/04 Gateway East, Singapore 189721, Singapore

If disposing of this product, please recycle the paper.

Preface

Renal anemia is one of the most common complications in patients with chronic renal insufficiency. It not only affects the patient's quality of life but also induces high mortality and socioeconomic burden. In the past few decades, the treatment of renal anemia has been significantly shaped by the emergence of human recombinant erythropoietin and iron supplements, the former is also called as erythropoietin-stimulating agents (ESAs). They significantly reduced the requirement for blood transfusions, consequently improving patients' quality of life. Despite the use of high-dose ESAs, many patients still face significant clinical challenges, including difficulty in achieving target hemoglobin levels. On the other hand, the inconvenience of ESAs as an injective form also restricts their use for nondialysis patients. More importantly, a number of patients with renal anemia are hyporesponsive to ESA therapy and even develop pure red cell dysplasia (PRCA). All of these tough clinical situations of renal anemia are also called refractory renal anemia. Such unmet clinical needs are really challenging issues for both physicians and patients. Fortunately, with the rapid progress of technology, we are continuously witnessing the emergence of innovative drugs for renal anemia, which are able to help doctors overcome this tough clinical challenge. Specifically, the advent of hypoxia-inducible factor proline-hydroxylase inhibitors (HIF-PHI), a novel revolutionary drug for renal anemia, has substantially demonstrated its unique efficacy in the treatment of this disease through a number of solid clinical trials.

This book collected 33 interesting cases with quite complex clinical experience during their journeys to treat renal anemia. We are pleased to share with readers many interesting and unique cases from various regions of China, which indeed partly reflects our experience based on clinical practice. And I believe, though the case may just be the case, but it does enlighten the doctor to have a new idea when they come across a complex situation. In these interesting cases, we are happy to envisage the unique role of HIF-PHI, roxadustat, which played a critical role in the treatment of these difficult cases of renal anemia. This experience has really enriched our knowledge to this new type of drug and motivated us to further explore its potential in the future clinical practice.

Frankly speaking, as the case collection, there are definitely some limitations in its nature. Notably, the cases come from different hospitals, and physicians may have different practice habits or experiences. However, we highly value the spirit they demonstrate when facing puzzling and thorny cases. And the successful stories for these cases inspire us to put them together to share with our colleagues for their critics and comments, which I believe will be helpful to improve our clinical practice in combating against renal anemia.

Finally, I would like to extend my gratitude to all the authors who contributed their valuable cases and wisdom in treating complicated renal anemia. I would like to express my sincere appreciation to Dr. Neeraja Padmanabhan and Springer Nature for their kind assistance in publishing this book.

Nanjing, China   Bi-Cheng Liu

Contents

Editors and Contributors

Editor

Bi-Cheng Liu Institute of Nephrology, Zhongda Hospital, Southeast University Nanjing China

Associate Editor

Bin Wang Department of Nephrology Zhongda Hospital, Southeast University Nanjing China

Contributors

Weijing Bian

Wen-Xiu Chang

Li Chen

Xiaonong Chen

Hong Cheng

Hong Chu

Chunli-Cui

Jiaxiang Ding

Jie Dong

Yinke Du

Xiao Fu

Liangying Gan

Chenni Gao

Zhu-Mei Gao

Leyi Gu

Da-Qing Hong

Jing Hu

Rong-rong Hu

Han-Wei Huang

Hong-Li Jiang

Ming-Zhu Li

Minxia Li

Xue-mei Li

Yuehong Li

Zuo-Lin Li

Xiao-Wan Liang

Dong-Wei Liu

Hong Liu

Jia-Feng Liu

Jie Liu

Xiao Liu

XiaoMing Liu

Ying-Hong Liu

Zhangsuo Liu

Zhang-Suo Liu

Renhua Lu

Jiayi Lv

Kun-Ling Ma

Xiaofei Man

Zhiguo Mao

Li-Jun Mou

San-Tao Ou

Huihua Pang

Panai Song

Lin Sun

Ri-Ning Tang

Bin Wang

Feng-Mei Wang

Hai-yun Wang

Pei Wang

Rong Wang

Tao Wang

Wei Wang

Min Wu

Gong Xiao

Xiang-Cheng Xiao

Kewei Xie

Xiaoyu Xie

Yan-Yun Xie

Hui Xu

Xiaoyi Xu

Yan Xu

Jun Xue

Yan-Tu

Qinghua Yang

Xiaowei Yang

Li Yao

Mu-Yao Ye

Qing Yin

Li You

Chen-Yu

Feng Yu

Qiong-Jing Yuan

Hao Zhang

LiHong Zhang

Mo Zhang

Wei-Wei Zhang

Wen Zheng

Hong-Shan Zhou

Huizi Zhu

Nan Zhu

Xin-Wang Zhu

Zhen Zhuang

Yang Zou

Li Zuo

Part I

ESA Hyporesponsive CKD Anemia

The advent of erythropoietin-stimulating agents (ESAs) has led to a significant progress in the treatment of renal anemia, which has largely reduced the need for blood transfusion. However, the rate for reaching hemoglobin target is still not as ideal as expected even though ESAs have been well prescribed. It is commonly called ESA hyporesponsiveness. Although the exact incidence of ESA hyporesponsiveness remains unclear, it is well recognized that this linical issue is closely associated with a poor prognosis and high risk of death, and which causes a great challenge for clinical practice. The causes of ESA hyporesponsiveness are diverse, which include but are not limited to iron deficiency, hyperparathyroidism, inflammatory or infectious status, increased C-reactive protein (CRP) levels, malnutrition, vitamin B12 or folic acid deficiency, and inadequate dialysis. These factors may act alone or in combination, leading to poor efficacy of ESAs. How to properly manage these special patient groups is an unmet clinical need. In this part, we present some cases of renal anemia with ESA hyporesponsiveness, covering both nondialysis and dialysis patients and providing references for managing this special group of patients.

Treatment of a Patient with Severe Anemia and Systemic Lupus Erythematosus

Kewei Xie, Huihua Pang, Renhua Lu, and Leyi Gu

1.1   Case Presentation

A 32-year-old female patient presented with persistent general fatigue, chest tightness, palpitations, and dizziness for 2 weeks. Prior to admission, she did not report any recognized causes for these symptoms. She denied experiencing any skin, oral, or nasal bleeding, fever, gastrointestinal distress, abdominal pain, diarrhea, erythema, joint pain, or any other discomfort. Routine blood tests revealed abnormal values, including a hemoglobin level of 60 g/L, red blood cell count of $2.5 \times 10^{1-2}$/L, white blood cell count of 3.8×10^9/L, and platelet count of 148×10^9/L. The patient had a past medical history of systemic lupus erythematosus and lupus nephritis (class III) and was currently receiving treatment with 10 mg prednisone daily, 0.1 g hydroxychloroquine twice daily, and 100 mg aspirin daily.

The postadmission renal function test revealed notable elevations in urea (18.90 mmol/L), creatinine (382.0 μmol/L), and uric acid (453.00 μmol/L), accompanied by a high cysteine protease inhibitor C level (3.91 mg/L). The estimated glomerular filtration rate (eGFR, EPI) was 10 mL/min, and the total 24-h urinary protein concentration was 383.4 mg. Urine analysis revealed urinary protein ± and hematuria with a microscopic red blood cell count of 29.1/HPF, while the white blood cell count was 1.4/HPF. Her routine blood examination revealed a white blood cell count of 4.47×10^9/L, with 74.3% neutrophils. Hemoglobin levels had decreased to 55 g/L, which is indicative of severe anemia, whereas the platelet count was 220×10^9/L, and the reticulocyte count was 0.026. The patient's albumin level was low at 30.4 g/L, and her erythropoietin (EPO) level was 7.80 IU/L. Folic acid and vitamin B12 levels were normal. Complement C3 was 0.82 g/L, and complement C4 was 0.27 g/L. The testing also revealed that the titer of anti-dsDNA

K. Xie · H. Pang (✉) · R. Lu (✉) · L. Gu (✉)
Department of Nephrology, Molecular Cell Laboratory for Kidney Disease, Shanghai Peritoneal Dialysis Research Center, Uremia Diagnosis and Treatment Center, Ren Ji Hospital, Shanghai Jiao Tong University School of Medicine, Shanghai, China

© The Author(s) 2025
B.-C. Liu (ed.), *Treatment of Refractory Renal Anemia*,
https://doi.org/10.1007/978-981-97-7636-8_1

antibodies was 22.24 IU/ml, and the titer of antinuclear antibodies was 1:160. Anti-neutrophil cytoplasmic antibody titers were negative, and no significant abnormalities were noted in other biochemical tests. Tests related to hemolytic anemia also returned negative results. Imaging and electrocardiogram examinations revealed no significant abnormalities.

The assessment of renal function indicated that the patient's kidney dysfunction had reached stage 5, with a poor renal structure by kidney ultrasound detection. Additionally, we identified severe iron deficiency in this patient, manifesting as significantly reduced levels of serum iron, total iron-binding capacity, and ferritin (serum iron: 5.9 μmol/L; total iron-binding capacity: 35.80 μmol/L; ferritin: 97.00 μg/L; and soluble transferrin receptor: 26.31 nmol/L). Despite the patient's history of systemic lupus erythematosus, her lupus activity was not significant, with a Systemic Lupus Erythematosus Disease Activity Index (SLEDAI) score of less than 4. For this patient, our treatment plan entailed iron supplementation, which began with intravenous iron administration of 100 mg for 5 consecutive days, followed by daily oral iron supplementation with ferrous succinate at a dose of 200 mg. Regular hemodialysis was scheduled three times per week, and the patient also received EPO injections once weekly, with each injection containing 10,000 units. After a 3-month follow-up period, we observed a significant increase in the patient's ferritin, serum iron, and total iron-binding capacity. However, her hemoglobin levels remained consistently below 100 g/L, and regular assessments indicated no significant lupus disease activity. Given these findings, we believe that the combination of erythropoietin and iron supplementation had reached its therapeutic limit in this patient, and further benefits were unlikely.

During the third month of follow-up, to achieve the patient's hemoglobin targets, we modified the anemia treatment plan to incorporate oral roxadustat. Accounting for the patient's weight (55 kg) and her current hemoglobin status, we initiated a dosage of 70 mg three times weekly and concomitantly discontinued oral iron supplementation. After 1 month of this revised treatment, the patient's hemoglobin levels significantly improved, surpassing the target value and exceeding 110 g/L. Notably, this increase in hemoglobin did not significantly affect the patient's serum iron level, total iron-binding capacity, or ferritin level.

The patients' hemoglobin levels are shown in Fig. 1.1.

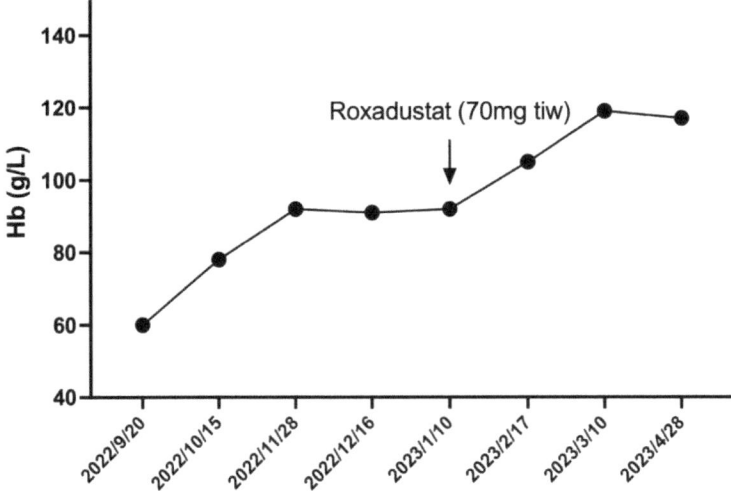

Fig. 1.1   Changes in hemoglobin levels

1.2   Discussion

A young female patient presented with severe anemia. Upon biochemical and imaging evaluations, it was discovered that she was in the end stage of kidney disease. Additionally, her medical history included systemic lupus erythematosus and severe iron deficiency, which complicated the identification of the specific cause of her anemia. After excluding lupus as the primary cause of her anemia, we included iron and erythropoietin in her treatment plan. Despite a notable improvement in her anemia status after 3 months of therapy, the desired outcome was not achieved, and her hemoglobin levels remained below the target range. Intriguingly, during this period, her serum iron concentration increased significantly, and her hemoglobin levels rose but remained below 110 g/L. Consequently, we adjusted her medication regimen, and within 1 month of taking roxadustat orally, her hemoglobin levels increased substantially, reaching the target range.

After thorough assessment, it became evident that for this particular patient, the primary cause of her anemia was chronic kidney failure rather than systemic lupus erythematosus. However, the following question remains: why did treatment with EPO yield unsatisfactory results for this patient, whereas roxadustat successfully helped her obtain an optimal hemoglobin level?

The kidneys are vital not only for eliminating metabolic waste and excess water from the body and regulating acid–base balance but also as endocrine organs of utmost importance [1–2]. EPO, formally referred to as erythropoietin, which is synthesized by the kidneys, is a naturally occurring human glycoprotein hormone that has potent stimulatory effects on erythropoiesis [3]. Clinically, recombinant human EPO is administered to patients suffering from anemia associated with renal insufficiency [4–5], triggering a cascade of events in the bone marrow and encouraging the continuous production of red blood cells to compensate for the functionality lost by aging red blood cells[6–8]. However, the efficacy of EPO on hematopoiesis in patients can be influenced by numerous factors. When administering EPO, it is crucial to consider the nutritional status of the patient, the presence of iron deficiency, infections, other immune-related diseases, or any other contributing factors [9–11]. Moreover, patients often exhibit varying responses to EPO, ranging from strong sensitivity to suboptimal responses. Furthermore, EPO may result in a rare yet critical side effect, namely, anti-EPO antibody-mediated pure red cell aplasia (PRCA) [12]. Additionally, resistance to EPO is common in 20–40% of patients treated, probably due to functional iron deficiency, reflecting the difficulties in managing iron deficiency associated with the chronic inflammation resulting from CKD [13]. In this patient, we were unable to definitively exclude the presence of EPO antibodies and EPO resistance.

EPO, which is the pivotal regulator of erythroid differentiation, is intricately modulated by hypoxia-inducible factor (HIF). Among the HIF isoforms, HIF2α appears to be the chief orchestrator of EPO transcription, although HIF1α and 3α may exert additional influences on erythroid maturation [14]. Moreover, HIF plays a critical role in the regulation of iron, a fundamental component of erythropoiesis[15]. HIF facilitates this regulation by inducing the synthesis of proteins involved in iron management, thereby ensuring sufficient iron availability for hematopoiesis [16]. Iron is a crucial component of hemoglobin and plays a significant role in erythrocyte differentiation, proliferation, and the regulation of HIF itself [17]. Renal anemia arises when there is a deficit in EPO synthesis stimulation due to reduced HIF expression. Thus, to address this, HIF prolyl hydroxylase inhibitors (HIF-PHIs) stabilize HIF, enabling its potent function even under normoxic conditions [18]. Consequently, unlike conventional erythropoiesis-stimulating agents, HIF-PHIs can increase iron absorption from the intestine and augment the iron supply from reticuloendothelial macrophages and hepatocytes into the plasma, increasing the availability of iron for hematopoiesis [19]. Roxadustat is the sole HIF-PHI marketed globally. Clinical studies in Japan and China have revealed that HIF-PHIs not only stimulate hematopoiesis but also reduce hepcidin, which is the key regulator of iron metabolism, and increase total iron-binding capacity (TIBC), a measure of iron transport capacity [20]. This multifaceted approach holds promise in the management of conditions associated with erythropoiesis and iron metabolism [21]. For our patient, decreased transferrin receptor activity and impaired iron utilization could explain why her response to rosuvastatin was more favorable than that to EPO. Research suggests that patients with uremia and SLE tend to maintain a prolonged inflammatory state. This condition effectively modulates the degradation of ferritin-mediated iron transport channels, ultimately sequestering iron in the form of ferritin within the cells of the reticuloendothelial system. As a result, the sequestered iron cannot be utilized for hemoglobin production, which subsequently explains the presence of anemia in these patients [22].

In conclusion, we present the case of a patient with stage 5 chronic kidney disease coupled with systemic lupus erythematosus. Initially, despite iron supplementation and treatment with EPO, the patient's anemia improved only partially, failing to reach the desired hemoglobin target levels. However, after the patient's medication was transitioned to roxadustat, the targeted hemoglobin level was successfully attained. We speculate that the inability to achieve the hemoglobin target level despite iron supplementation could be attributed to decreased transferrin receptor activity and impaired iron utilization. In this context, roxadustat was determined to be superior in effectively managing the patient's anemia.

References

1. Groothof D, Bakker SJL. Evaluating the effect of bempedoic acid on kidney function: call for cautious implementation. Lancet Diabetes Endocrinol. 2024;12(4):228.
2. Ando T, Miura K, Yabuuchi T, Shirai Y, Ishizuka K, Kanda S, Harita Y, Hirasawa K, Hamada R, Ishikura K, Inoue E, Hattori M. Long-term kidney function of Lowe syndrome: a nationwide study of pediatric and adult patients. Nephrol Dial Transplant. 2024;31:gfae080.
3. Kobayashi H, Davidoff O, Pujari-Palmer S, Drevin M, Haase VH. EPO synthesis induced by HIF-PHD inhibition is dependent on myofibroblast transdifferentiation and colocalizes with non-injured nephron segments in murine kidney fibrosis. Acta Physiol (Oxf). 2022;235(4):e13826.
4. Sebestyén MG, Hegge JO, Noble MA, Lewis DL, Herweijer H, Wolff JA. Progress toward a nonviral gene therapy protocol for the treatment of anemia. Hum Gene Ther. 2007;18(3):269–85.
5. Martí-Carvajal AJ, Agreda-Pérez LH, Solà I, Simancas-Racines D. Erythropoiesis-stimulating agents for anemia in rheumatoid arthritis. Cochrane Database Syst Rev. 2013;2013(2):CD000332.
6. Benderro GF, LaManna JC. Kidney EPO expression during chronic hypoxia in aged mice. Adv Exp Med Biol. 2013;765:9–14.
7. Lu Z, Lu F, Zhang R, Guo S. Interaction between anemia and hyperuricemia in the risk of all-cause mortality in patients with chronic kidney disease. Front Endocrinol (Lausanne). 2024;15:1286206.
8. Kremer D, Knobbe TJ, Vinke JSJ, Groothof D, Post A, Annema C, Abrahams AC, van Jaarsveld BC, de Borst MH, Berger SP, TransplantLines Investigators, SJL B, Eisenga MF. Iron deficiency, anemia, and patient-reported outcomes in kidney transplant recipients. Am J Transplant. 2024;S1600–6135(24):00213–2.
9. Ding X, Sun S, Zhang J, Zhao H, Lun F, Liu X, Zhen Y, Dong J, Wu J. Ferric citrate for the treatment of hyperphosphatemia and iron deficiency anaemia in patients with NDD-CKD: a systematic review and meta-analysis. Front Pharmacol. 2024;15:1285012.
10. D'Alessandro A, Krisnevskaya E, Leguizamon V, Hernández I, de la Torre C, Bech JJ, Navarro JT, Vives-Corrons JL. SARS-CoV-2 infection and anemia-a focus on RBC deformability and membrane proteomics-integrated observational prospective study. Microorganisms. 2024;12(3):453.
11. Zhang X, Gao BX, Guo CY, Su T. A 71-year-old male with a life-threatening recurrence of hemolytic anemia, thrombocytopenia, and acute kidney injury after pembrolizumab therapy: a case report. BMC Geriatr. 2023;23(1):478.
12. Wu Y, Cai X, Ni J, Lin X. Resolution of epoetin-induced pure red cell aplasia, successful re-challenge with roxadustat. Int J Lab Hematol. 2020;42(6):e291–3.
13. Elliott J. Therapeutics of managing reduced red cell mass associated with chronic kidney disease—is there a case for earlier intervention? J Vet Pharmacol Ther. 2023;46(3):145–57.
14. Ogawa C, Tsuchiya K, Maeda K. Hypoxia-inducible factor Prolyl hydroxylase inhibitors and iron metabolism. Int J Mol Sci. 2023;24(3):3037.
15. Fan J, Lei W, Wang L, Ge W. A nomogram for predicting the risk of treatment failure of roxadustat in peritoneal dialysis with renal anemia. Sci Rep. 2024;14(1):7622.

16. Tanaka H, Tani A, Onoda T, Ishii T. Hypoxia-inducible factor Prolyl hydroxylase inhibitors and hypothyroidism: an analysis of the Japanese Pharmacovigilance database. In Vivo. 2024;38(2):917–22.
17. Ganz T, Locatelli F, Arici M, Akizawa T, Reusch M. Iron parameters in patients treated with Roxadustat for anemia of chronic kidney disease. J Clin Med. 2023;12(13):4217.
18. Chen H, Cheng Q, Wang J, Zhao X, Zhu S. Long-term efficacy and safety of hypoxia-inducible factor prolyl hydroxylase inhibitors in anaemia of chronic kidney disease: a meta-analysis including 13,146 patients. J Clin Pharm Ther. 2021;46(4):999–1009.
19. Tan W, Wang X, Sun Y, Wang X, He J, Zhong L, Jiang X, Sun Y, Tian E, Li Z, He L, Hao Y, Tang B, Hua W, Ma X, Yang J. Roxadustat reduces left ventricular mass index compared to rHuEPO in haemodialysis patients in a randomized controlled trial. J Intern Med. 2024;295(5):620–33.
20. Chen N, Hao C, Liu BC, Lin H, Wang C, Xing C, Liang X, Jiang G, Liu Z, Li X, Zuo L, Luo L, Wang J, Zhao MH, Liu Z, Cai GY, Hao L, Leong R, Wang C, Liu C, Neff T, Szczech L, Yu KP. Roxadustat treatment for anemia in patients undergoing long-term dialysis. N Engl J Med. 2019;381(11):1011–22.
21. Li H, Hu SM, Li YM, Ciancio G, Tadros NN, Tao Y, Bai YJ, Shi YY. Beneficial effect of roxadustat on early posttransplant anemia and iron utilization in kidney transplant recipients: a retrospective comparative cohort study. Ann Transl Med. 2022;10(24):1360.
22. Vanarsa K, Ye Y, Han J, Xie C, Mohan C, Wu T. Inflammation associated anemia and ferritin as disease markers in SLE. Arthritis Res Ther. 2012;14(4):R182.

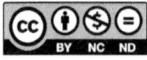

Treatment of a Hemodialysis Patient with Renal Anemia Complicated By Gastrointestinal Bleeding

2

Yinke Du and Li Yao

2.1 Case Presentation

A 73-year-old male patient was admitted to hospital with renal insufficiency for four years and shortness of breath for six days. Four years before admission, his urine test shows proteinuria 2+, occult blood 1+, and urine microalbumin (MA) exceeded 1000 mg/L. Continuous oral medication was administered to decrease serum creatinine and reduce urinary protein excretion. Six days prior to admission, the patient experienced chest tightness, shortness of breath in the morning, and occasional chest pain and was able to lie flat at night. His serum creatinine increased to 597 μmol/L; his hemoglobin reached 91 g/L, and transferrin saturation was 15%. Ferritin was 290 ug/L, and BNP was 855 pg/mL. He was then diagnosed with chronic kidney disease (CKD) stage 5, diabetic nephropathy stage 5, renal anemia, hypertension, coronary heart disease, and left heart failure. During hospitalization, the patient developed shortness of breath and melena, and his Hb decreased to 42 g/L (Fig. 2.1). The patient was diagnosed with upper gastrointestinal bleeding in the Department of Gastroenterology and received treatment with gastroscopic hemostasis and blood transfusion. Simultaneously, maintenance hemodialysis (three times a week) was initiated. After half a month of treatment, symptoms improved. BNP decreased to 620 pg/mL, and Hb increased to 80 g/L after transfusion (Fig. 2.1). After discharge, the patient continued to undergo regular hemodialysis treatment and regular follow-up in our hospital. The transferrin saturation ranged from 14 to 25%; the ferritin was 220–560 μg/L; the albumin was 30–36 g/L, and CRP, IL-6, procalcitonin, folic acid, and B12 were within the normal range. Recombinant human erythropoietin (rHuEPO) was 12,000–16,000 units per week. Sucrose iron was 200–300 mg per month, but the Hb level fluctuated between 80 and 83 g/L. The patient had poor intake of meat and other proteins after

Y. Du · L. Yao (✉)
The First Hospital of China Medical University, Shenyang, China

HGB (g/l)

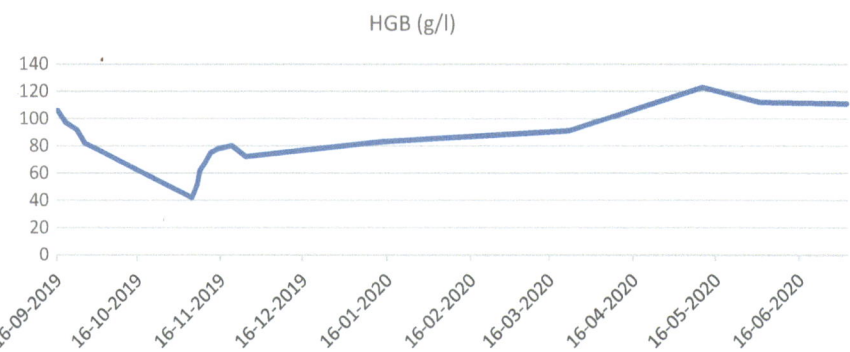

Fig. 2.1 Changes of hemoglobin levels with the time in the patient

gastrointestinal bleeding. He was given 100 mg of roxadustat orally once weekly, and regular follow-up continued. Six months after the treatment of roxadustat, the patient's Hb rose to 123 g/L, and the subsequent follow-up showed stability between 110 and 120 g/L. The patient is still undergoing regular hemodialysis therapy.

The patient had a history of diabetes for over 20 years and achieved better blood sugar control through oral medications. The patient also suffered from hypertension for 15 years, with blood pressure ranging from 160–220/85–110 mmHg (1 mmHg = 0.133 kPa). Nifedipine controlled-release tablets, 30 mg orally once daily, were prescribed, but blood pressure control was inadequate.

2.2 Discussion

Besides iron supplementation for the treatment of renal anemia, ESA is also of great significance and widely utilized in the clinical setting. Nevertheless, the response to ESA might be insufficient, particularly in instances of iron deficiency and inflammation. Patients with low responsiveness to ESA require higher doses of EPO and iron, but it is still challenging to achieve consistent Hb standards, and the clinical prognosis is deemed unfavorable. Roxadustat is a new-generation hypoxia-inducing factor prolyl hydroxylase inhibitor (HIF-PHI), which can comprehensively regulate erythropoiesis and solve renal anemia among dialysis patients. Additionally, roxadustat can significantly enhance the binding affinity of transferrin and total iron, reduce transferrin saturation (TSAT), and maintain serum iron and Hb levels without any variation in the dose of roxadustat under the circumstance of non-routine intravenous iron supplementation [1]. In contrast, the effect of EPO on Hb is inhibited by inflammation. Hence, dialysis patients need significantly higher doses of EPO. Inflammation has a negligible impact on the efficacy of roxadustat. Research studies have indicated that roxadustat can also contribute in reducing the levels of micro-inflammatory cytokines and has a superior safety profile [2]. Therefore, in the treatment of renal anemia, roxadustat is effective in alleviating clinical symptoms such as pale complexion, fatigue, palpitation, shortness of breath and improving cardiac function and quality of life. Roxadustat can also reduce the inflammatory response of patients and has a beneficial effect in the clinical management of renal anemia. Since the Hb level of this patient did not reach the target range, it was suspected that the patient might have low ESA responsiveness. There are two types of hyporesponsiveness to ESA: initial ESA low response and acquired ESA low response. Low ESA responsiveness is defined as no increase in Hb levels from the baseline after 1 month of treatment with an appropriate dose of ESA based on the patient's body weight. Acquired ESA low reactivity is defined as increasing the ESA dose by more than 50% of the stable dose to maintain Hb stability after a stable ESA treatment. The causes of ESA hyporeactivity involve iron deficiency, concomitant inflammatory diseases, chronic blood loss, hyperparathyroidism, osteitis fibrosis, aluminum poisoning, hemoglobinopathy, malignant tumors, malnutrition, hemolysis, inadequate dialysis, the use of angiotensin-converting enzyme inhibitors (ACEI) or angiotensin-II receptor antagonists (ARB), hyplenism, and recombinant human erythropoietin (rHuEPO) antibody-mediated pure red cell dysplasia (PRCA). Among them, iron deficiency is the most prevalent [3], but in this case, we speculate that the patient has been experiencing malnutrition following gastrointestinal bleeding. Besides the common factors like inflammation and iron deficiency, malnutrition is frequently overlooked. Therefore, while correcting renal anemia, we should also pay attention to the patient's diet and albumin level.

References

1. Chen N, Hao C, Liu BC, et al. Roxadustat treatment for anemia in patients undergoing long-term dialysis. N Engl J Med. 2019;381(11):1011–22.
2. Teng F, Li XM. Hypoxia-inducible factor and renal anemia. Chin J Nephrol. 2017;33(1):63–8.
3. Expert group on diagnosis and treatment of renal anemia CSoN. Chinese expert consensus on diagnosis and treatment of renal anemia. Chin J Nephrol. 2018;34(11):860–6.

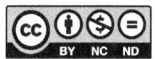

Roxadustat on Renal Anemia in Patients with Maintenance Hemodialysis

Zhu-Mei Gao and Hong-Li Jiang

3.1 Case Presentation

A 61-year-old male patient was admitted to the Affiliated Hospital of Xi'an Jiaotong Medical University in July 2015 due to blurred vision. A detailed examination revealed a hemoglobin level of 96 g/L, a blood urea nitrogen level of 19 mmol/L, a creatinine level of 504 μmol/L, and a uric acid level of 576 μmol/L. Meanwhile, ultrasound results revealed bilateral polycystic kidneys and a polycystic liver. He was then diagnosed with "polycystic kidney, chronic kidney disease stage 4, renal anemia, and polycystic liver" and received a subcutaneous injection of recombinant human erythropoietin (r-HuEPO) at a dose of 10,000 IU once a week for anemia but was not followed up regularly.

In August 2016, he presented at our hospital due to malaise. Laboratory examinations revealed his blood urea nitrogen level was 32.48 mmol/L, serum creatinine level 886 μmol/L, and hemoglobin level 82 g/L. Serological test results for tumor markers and ANA, anti-double-stranded DNA, anti-glomerular basement membrane, and anti-neutrophilic cytoplasmic antibodies were negative and so as the results for hepatitis B and C or HIV infections. The patient was diagnosed with chronic kidney disease stage 5 due to worsening symptoms and significantly elevated serum toxin levels. During this hospitalization, he started receiving thrice-weekly hemodialysis after the arteriovenous fistula was established. The patient continued to receive subcutaneous injections of r-HuEPO at a weekly dose of 10,000 IU for anemia, but was not stable, and his hemoglobin concentrations fluctuated between 82 g/L and 101 g/L.

In April 2021, upon re-examination, the hemoglobin level was 80 g/L. Thus, his medication regimen was switched to roxadustat at a dosage of 120 mg three times per week. Two months later, the patient's hemoglobin level returned to normal at

Z.-M. Gao · H.-L. Jiang (✉)

Department of Nephrology Hospital, The First Affiliated Hospital of Xi'an Jiaotong University, Xi'an, Shanxi, China

© The Author(s) 2025

B.-C. Liu (ed.), *Treatment of Refractory Renal Anemia*,

https://doi.org/10.1007/978-981-97-7636-8_3

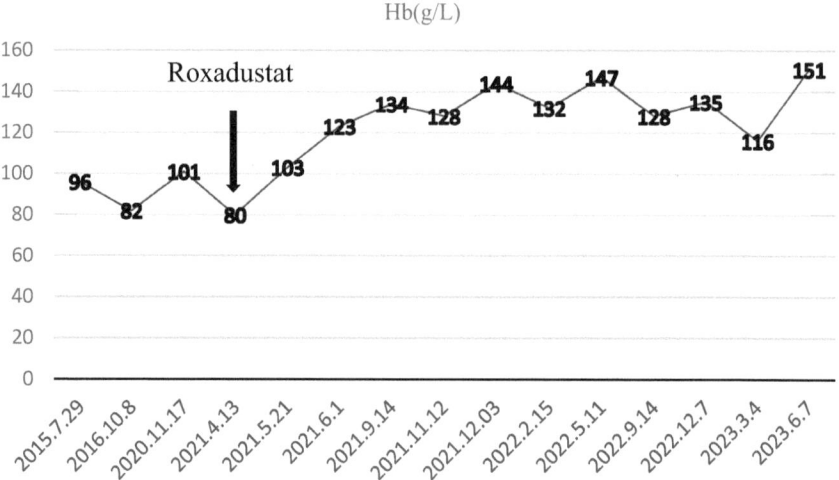

Fig. 3.1 Changes in patient's hemoglobin levels

123 g/L. During the 2-year follow-up, the patient's hemoglobin levels were maintained at a normal level, while the roxadustat dosage was gradually reduced to 20 mg three times per week. The most recent hemoglobin concentration was 151 g/L; therefore, roxadustat was stopped (Fig. 3.1).

He had a 7-year history of hypertension, with a maximum blood pressure of 180/110 mmHg. Initially, he took Nifedipine Controlled-Release Tablets, 30mg twice daily to control his blood pressure, which was maintained at around 120/80 mmHg, and there was no need for antihypertensive drugs now. Physical examination revealed a chronically ill appearance and no pitting edema in either lower limbs. He had no significant iron deficiency (iron, 26.6 μmol/L; transferrin saturation, 53.3%; and ferritin, 265 ~ 590 μg/L).

3.2   Discussion

This middle-aged male patient on regular hemodialysis presented with moderate anemia, and he accepted a sufficient dosage of EPO, which was initially effective, but his hemoglobin decreased later. Then, the patient's medication regimen was switched from EPO to roxadustat, and the dosage of roxadustat was adjusted according to the instructions. Surprisingly, his hemoglobin level was maintained between 120 g/L and 130 g/L; therefore, it was possible to discontinue the use of EPO or roxadustat.

Renal anemia is a common complication of chronic kidney disease (CKD), and the main treatment options is erythropoiesis-stimulating agents (ESAs), but erythropoietin hyporesponsiveness can also come with it. In clinical practice, adjusting the dose or frequency of administration of ESAs often used to solve this problem. However, using higher ESA doses to achieve higher hemoglobin levels is not beneficial and is associated with a greater risk of death and cardiovascular outcomes in hemodialysis patients [1, 2]. Thus, it is necessary to find new ways to improve renal anemia when patients have a poor hematopoietic response to ESAs.

Several hypoxia-inducible factor prolyl hydroxylase inhibitors (HIF-PHIs) can be used as an alternative, of which roxadustat is the first approved for clinical use for the treatment of renal anemia. Emerging evidence suggests that roxadustat may be beneficial for patients who inadequately respond to ESAs. Roxadustat effectively ameliorates anemia in patients with CKD by stabilizing HIF-α subunits, promoting endogenous EPO production, improving iron metabolism and upregulating EPO receptor expression [3]. A single-center, prospective investigation of dialysis patients with erythropoietin hyporesponsiveness found that significant anti-anemia effects could be achieved in most patients with erythropoietin hyporesponsiveness after treatment with roxadustat [4]. Moreover, another study conducted a systematic review and network meta-analysis of RCTs comparing HIF-PHIs versus ESAs, which indicated that there were no notable differences in the risk of cardiovascular events, hyperkalemia, cancer, pneumonia, upper respiratory tract infection, nasopharyngitis, urinary tract infection, hypotension, and muscle spasms between HIF-PHIs and ESAs for treating anemia in dialysis patients [5]. Roxadustat can -reduce total cholesterol and low-density lipoprotein (LDL) cholesterol levels as well. Thus, roxadustat has a significant impact on improving the anemia status in CKD patients who are unresponsive to ESAs.

Iron supplementation is another major traditional treatment for anemia in patients with CKD. However, its absorption and retention must be strictly controlled due to its high toxicity. A meta-analysis including 20 studies with 14,737 participants demonstrated that there was no significant difference in the effect on transferrin saturation or ferritin between HIF-PHIs and ESAs, but compared with ESAs, HIF-PHIs significantly increased the iron, total iron-binding capacity, and transferrin levels [6]. Therefore, unlike ESAs, HIF-PHIs may increase iron absorption from the intestinal tract and iron supply from reticuloendothelial macrophages and hepatocytes into the plasma, thereby facilitating the availability of iron for hematopoiesis [7].

In addition, roxadustat reduces serum cholesterol and triglyceride levels in both dialysis-dependent and dialysis-independent patients with CKD, which is deemed beneficial for the cardiovascular and cerebrovascular systems [8, 9]. The study also showed that decreased levels of phospholipids, lysophospholipids, and sphingolipid metabolism were correlated with the improvement of anemia after roxadustat treatment in peritoneal dialysis patients [10].

An inflammatory state is one of the most frequent causes of ESA resistance in CKD patients. For example, patients with high C-reactive protein (CRP) levels were shown to require significantly higher ESA doses to achieve comparable hemoglobin levels even after controlling for potential confounding variables [11]. However, roxadustat led to similar hemoglobin responses in patients with high CRP levels and those with normal CRP levels [4, 12]. These studies suggested that inflammation has little effect on the erythropoiesis effect of roxadustat. In addition, it has been reported that the administration of roxadustat significantly increases CD73 synthesis but suppresses the activation of the AIM2 inflammasome in ischemia–reperfusion-induced acute kidney injury [13]. This trial confirmed that roxadustat has a potential anti-inflammatory effect, but more clinical studies are needed to confirm this possibility.

In conclusion, roxadustat is determined as an effective treatment for renal anemia in both nondialysis-dependent and dialysis-dependent CKD patients. The effects of roxadustat in treating renal anemia are multifaceted and include promoting endogenous EPO production and facilitating serum transferrin levels, as well as intestinal iron absorption, reducing the level of hepcidin, and adjusting the lipid metabolism.

Here, we reported the case of a dialysis-dependent CKD patient with anemia who had a poor response to high-dose ESAs in the fifth year of treatment. Then, the patient's medication regimen was switched from ESAs to roxadustat, and the dosage of roxadustat was adjusted according to the instructions. Finally, a normal range of hemoglobin levels could be maintained without the use of anemia-correcting drugs. In conclusion, roxadustat could effectively correct anemia. This case provides unique insights into the use of this new class of drug for treating patients who are resistant to ESAs.

References

1. Zhang Y, Thamer M, Kaufman JS, Cotter DJ, Hernán MA. High doses of epoetin do not lower mortality and cardiovascular risk among elderly hemodialysis patients with diabetes. Kidney Int. 2011;80(6):663–9.
2. Pérez-García R, Varas J, Cives A, et al. Increased mortality in haemodialysis patients administered high doses of erythropoiesis-stimulating agents: a propensity score-matched analysis. Nephrol Dial Transplant. 2018;33(4):690–9.
3. Kaplan JM, Sharma N, Dikdan S. Hypoxia-inducible factor and its role in the management of anemia in chronic kidney disease. Int J Mol Sci. 2018;19(2):389.
4. Zhou Y, Chen XX, Zhang YF, Lou JZ, Yuan HB. Roxadustat for dialysis patients with erythropoietin hypo-responsiveness: a single-center, prospective investigation. Intern Emerg Med. 2021;16(8):2193–9.
5. Chen D, Niu Y, Liu F, et al. Safety of HIF prolyl hydroxylase inhibitors for anemia in dialysis patients: a systematic review and network meta-analysis. Front Pharmacol. 2023;14:1163908.
6. Zheng Q, Zhang P, Yang H, et al. Effects of hypoxia-inducible factor prolyl hydroxylase inhibitors versus erythropoiesis-stimulating agents on iron metabolism and inflammation in patients undergoing dialysis: a systematic review and meta-analysis. Heliyon. 2023;9(4):e15310.
7. Ogawa C, Tsuchiya K, Maeda K. Hypoxia-inducible factor prolyl hydroxylase inhibitors and iron metabolism. Int J Mol Sci. 2023;24(3):3037.
8. Hirai K, Kaneko S, Minato S, et al. Effects of roxadustat on anemia, iron metabolism, and lipid metabolism in patients with non-dialysis chronic kidney disease. Front Med (Lausanne). 2023;10:1071342.
9. Csiky B, Schömig M, Esposito C, et al. Roxadustat for the maintenance treatment of anemia in patients with end-stage kidney disease on stable dialysis: a European phase 3, randomized, open-label, active-controlled study (PYRENEES). Adv Ther. 2021;38(10):5361–80.
10. Yang YH, Saimaiti Y, Zhao Y, Tang W. Plasma phospholipids profiling changes were associated with the therapeutic response to Roxadustat in peritoneal dialysis patients. Front Physiol. 2023;14:1279578.

11. Bradbury BD, Critchlow CW, Weir MR, Stewart R, Krishnan M, Hakim RH. Impact of elevated C-reactive protein levels on erythropoiesis- stimulating agent (ESA) dose and responsiveness in hemodialysis patients. Nephrol Dial Transplant. 2009;24(3):919–25.

12. Akizawa T, Iwasaki M, Yamaguchi Y, Majikawa Y, Reusch M. Phase 3, randomized, double-blind, active-comparator (Darbepoetin Alfa) study of oral roxadustat in CKD patients with anemia on hemodialysis in Japan. J Am Soc Nephrol. 2020;31(7):1628–39.

13. Yang H, Wu Y, Cheng M, et al. Roxadustat (FG-4592) protects against ischaemia-induced acute kidney injury via improving CD73 and decreasing AIM2 inflammasome activation. Nephrol Dial Transplant. 2023;38(4):858–75.

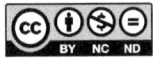

Treatment of Renal Anemia in a Peritoneal Dialysis Patient with Low Erythropoietic Response

4

Jing Hu and Hao Zhang

4.1 Case Presentation

The patient was 57-year-old man with high blood pressure and proteinuria for 17 years before admission. He was diagnosed with chronic glomerulonephritis by renal biopsy. He had elevated blood creatinine 10 years ago and entered stage 5 CKD 4 years ago, and he then received peritoneal dialysis. His dialysis dose was 8 L per day, and continuous ambulatory peritoneal dialysis (CAPD) was used. At the same time, human erythropoietin and oral iron were started to treat renal anemia. He underwent regular check-ups during dialysis treatment, and his hemoglobin fluctuated from 70 to 85 g/L. Six months before admission, the patient showed obvious dizziness and fatigue, and his hemoglobin was 56 g/L 3 months before admission. The patient was given a transfusion of concentrated red blood cells and stayed on rhu-EPO and iron; the dose of rhu-EPO was increased to 13,000 U/week, and his maximum hemoglobin concentration increased to 89 g/L. During follow-up observation after discharge, the patient's Hb gradually decreased, falling to a minimum of 61 g/L.

Physical examination on admission revealed weight 62 kg，BP 153/78 mmHg, chronic disease, anemia, clear breathing in both lungs, an enlarged left lower boundary of the heart, no jugular vein distention, and no edema of either lower limb.

Laboratory values were as follows: WBC, 6.8×10^9/L; RBC, 2.84×10^{12}/L; hemoglobin, 61 g/L; platelets, 108×10^9/ L; NT-proBNP, 5678 pg/ml; C-reactive protein, 5.6 mg/L; serum total protein, 56.3 g/L; albumin, 32.8 g/L; blood urea nitrogen, 24.5 mmol/L; creatinine, 956 μmol/L; serum calcium, 2.14 mmol/L; phosphorus, 2.84 mmol/L; uric acid, 523 μmol/L; and PTH, 820 pg/ml. Tests for tumor markers, autoantibodies (including anti-nuclear (anti-double-stranded DNA), anti-glomerular basement membrane, and anti-neutrophil antibodies), and viral infection

J. Hu · H. Zhang (✉)
Department of Nephrology, The Third Xiangya Hospital, Central South University, Changsha, China

© The Author(s) 2025
B.-C. Liu (ed.), *Treatment of Refractory Renal Anemia*,
https://doi.org/10.1007/978-981-97-7636-8_4

19

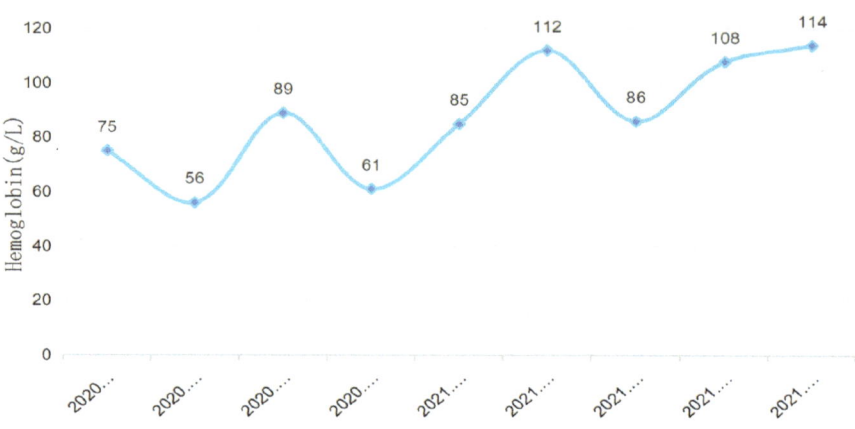

Fig. 4.1 Changes in hemoglobin levels

(hepatitis B and C or HIV infection) were all negative. Moreover, there was no evidence of hematologic disease (serum protein electrophoresis or immunofixation electrophoresis) or autoimmune hemolytic disease (Coombs test). The results indicated hyperphosphatemia and secondary hyperparathyroidism. The result of the peritoneal equilibrium test was 0.59, which was higher than that of the average transport type, with a total KT/V of 1.71, suggesting that solute clearance was sufficient.

The iron metabolism parameters included the following: ferritin, 653 ng/L; transferrin saturation, 17.3%; and total iron-binding capacity, 53 μmol/L. The patient did not have absolute iron deficiency but had low transferrin saturation and elevated ferritin, indicating iron transport disorder and relative iron deficiency.

The patient was treated with oral roxadustat 100 mg TIW and oral iron, and he received a low-phosphorus diet supplemented with an oral phosphorus binder and Cinacalcet to prevent hyperparathyroidism. His hemoglobin increased to 85 g/L 1 month after discharge and to 112 g/L 3 months later. Re-examination of iron metabolism parameters showed that ferritin decreased to 457 ng/L, transferrin saturation increased to 34%, and iPTH decreased to 432 pg/ml.

Six months after discharge, the patient discontinued roxadustat for financial reasons, and he switched to rhu-EPO 10,000 U subcutaneously once a week. However, hemoglobin decreased again to as low as 86 g/L. The patient returned to oral roxadustat 100 mg three times a week for 3 months earlier, after which the anemia gradually improved, and hemoglobin stabilized at 110–120 g/L at present (Fig. 4.1).

4.2   Discussion

This patient was a peritoneal dialysis patient with end-stage renal disease who had been on dialysis for 4 years. The patient took erythropoietin and iron to treat anemia for a long time, but his hemoglobin, which never reached the standard for anemia, was significantly aggravated after dialysis for about 3 years and could only be transiently improved by blood transfusion treatment. High-dose EPO and iron supplementation were still ineffective. His iron metabolism index suggested iron utilization disorder, relative iron deficiency, hyperphosphatemia, and secondary hyperparathyroidism. After switching to roxadustat, the patient's hemoglobin level steadily improved, reaching the treatment target of 110–130 g/L, and iron metabolism disorders and hyperparathyroidism have also improved. However, the patient discontinued roxadustat on his own; his anemia worsened after switching to rhu-EPO, but restarting roxadustat was still effective for anemia treatment.

Erythropoiesis-stimulating agents (ESAs) and iron agents have been the mainstays of treatment for renal anemia, but there remains an unmet clinical need due to the low response to ESAs in some patients. Although disease severity and comorbidities may partially contribute to the hyporeactivity of ESAs, the most common causes include iron deficiency, inflammation, secondary hyperparathyroidism, and dialysis insufficiency [1].

Solute clearance on dialysis in this patient was adequate, but the impairment of calcium and phosphorus metabolism, the presence of hyperphosphatemia, and secondary hyperparathyroidism combined with iron utilization disorders were likely responsible for the low response to erythropoietin (EPO) [2]. High doses of ESAs still do not meet the need for anemia treatment, and high doses of EPO increase the risk of cardiovascular events and even death [3, 4]. Therefore, finding new strategies to treat anemia in patients with hyporeactive ESAs remains to be an unmet need [5].

Roxadustat, a new-generation renal anemia drug with novel mechanisms, is an oral bioavailable hypoxia-inducible factor prolyl hydroxylase inhibitor that mimics the natural response to hypoxia [6]. Mechanistically, roxadustat not only promotes the production of endogenous EPO but also improves the absorption, transport, and utilization of iron and is not affected by inflammation, which is obviously different from the effects of ESAs, which can only supplement exogenous EPO [7, 8].

The patient had increased anemia after switching to EPO, but the anemia was corrected by roxadustat, indicating that roxadustat was continuously effective for treating low-response anemia in EPO patients.

Here, we report the case of a patient with renal anemia with a weak response to EPO due to hyperphosphatemia, secondary hyperparathyroidism, and iron utilization disorder who experienced effective and safe correction of anemia after two repeated administrations of roxadustat.

References

1. Wu HHL, Chinnadurai R. Erythropoietin-stimulating agent hyporesponsiveness in patients living with chronic kidney disease. Kidney Dis. 2022;8(2):103–14.
2. Tanaka M, Komaba H, Fukagawa M. Emerging association between parathyroid hormone and anemia in hemodialysis patients. Ther Apher Dial. 2018;22(3):242–5.
3. Batchelor EK, Kapitsinou P, Pergola PE, Kovesdy CP, Jalal DI. Iron deficiency in chronic kidney disease: updates on pathophysiology, diagnosis, and treatment. J Am Soc Nephrol. 2020;31(3):456–68.

4. Del Vecchio L, Locatelli F. An overview on safety issues related to erythropoiesis-stimulating agents for the treatment of anaemia in patients with chronic kidney disease. Expert Opin Drug Saf. 2016;15(8):1021–30.
5. Weir MR. Managing anemia across the stages of kidney disease in those hyporesponsive to erythropoiesis-stimulating agents. Am J Nephrol. 2021;52(6):450–66.
6. Haase VH. Hypoxia-inducible factor-prolyl hydroxylase inhibitors in the treatment of anemia of chronic kidney disease. Kidney Int Suppl. 2021;11(1):8–25.
7. Shih HM, Wu CJ, Lin SL. Physiology and pathophysiology of renal erythropoietin-producing cells. J Formos Med Assoc. 2018;117(11):955–63.
8. Zheng L, Tian J, Liu D, et al. Efficacy and safety of roxadustat for anaemia in dialysis-dependent and non-dialysis-dependent chronic kidney disease patients: a systematic review and meta-analysis. Br J Clin Pharmacol. 2021;88(3):919–32.

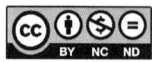

Treatment of Anemia in a Multiple Myeloma Patient with Deep Vein Thrombosis in the Lower Limb

5

Chenni Gao and Xiaonong Chen

5.1 Case Presentation

A 77-year-old female patient in good health was admitted to our department because of consistent fatigue and foamy urine in June 2019. These symptoms began 6 months earlier and were accompanied by increasing nocturia, dizziness, chest tightness, and shortness of breath. In May 2019, this patient was admitted to another hospital. Laboratory tests revealed a hemoglobin concentration of 76 g/L, urea nitrogen concentration of 22.4 mmol/L, creatinine concentration of 447 µmol/L, and 24-hour urinary protein concentration of 2.7 g. After seven cycles of intermittent hemodialysis, the patient's condition improved, and dialysis was stopped.

On June 13, 2019, the patient visited our outpatient department. A complete blood test revealed a hemoglobin concentration of 75 g/L, and abdominal ultrasound showed diffuse lesions in both kidneys (left kidney: 97 mm × 38 mm; right kidney: 100 mm × 41 mm). Her treatment regimen for anemia at that time was recombinant human erythropoietin (rHuEPO) (10,000 U) administered subcutaneously once a week. She was hospitalized for further therapy.

At admission, her temperature was 36.3 °C; pulse was 99 beats/minute; respiratory rate was 18 breaths/minute; blood pressure was 110/74 mmHg; height was 154.5 cm, and weight was 53 kg.

Laboratory results revealed the following: white blood cells 5.4×10^9/L, hemoglobin 64 g/L, platelets 112×10^9/L, total protein 67 g/L, albumin 35 g/L, urea nitrogen 31.7 mmol/L, creatinine 830 µmol/L, uric acid 575 µmol/L, triglyceride 1.5 mmol/L, total cholesterol 3.25 mmol/L, serum potassium 5.17 mmol/L, serum calcium 2.14 mmol/L, serum phosphorus 2.14 mmol/L, parathyroid hormone 145.8 pg/ml, and 25-hydroxyvitamin D3 58.99 nmol/L. Tests for antinuclear

C. Gao · X. Chen (✉)
Department of Nephrology, Ruijin Hospital, Shanghai Jiao Tong University School of Medicine, Shanghai, China
e-mail: cxn10419@rjh.com.cn

© The Author(s) 2025
B.-C. Liu (ed.), *Treatment of Refractory Renal Anemia*,
https://doi.org/10.1007/978-981-97-7636-8_5

23

antibodies, anti-glomerular basement membrane antibodies, and antineutrophil cytoplasmic antibodies were negative. Her immunoglobulin G was 6.63 g/L, immunoglobulin A 0.11 g/L, immunoglobulin M 0.07 g/L, immunoglobulin E 5 U/ml, blood free κ light chain 16.7 mg/L, blood free λ light chain >162 mg/L (κ/λ < 0.1), serum immunofixation electrophoresis λ (+), and urine immunofixation electrophoresis λ (+). Her 24-h urinary protein concentration was 4175 mg.

Etiologies for anemia included a negative fecal occult blood test, a serum iron concentration of 16.6 μmol/L, a transferrin concentration of 146 mg/dl, a total iron-binding capacity of 39.4 μmol/L, a transferrin saturation of 40.9%, a folic acid concentration of 12.26 ng/ml, and a vitamin B concentration of 12,249 pg/ml. Bone marrow aspirate smears revealed active bone marrow proliferation, a high granulocyte/erythrocyte ratio, active granulocyte proliferation, a right shift of the nucleus, and decreased erythroid hyperplasia. Mature red blood cells showed a rouleaux arrangement; megakaryocytic hyperplasia was still active; scattered small clusters of platelets were observed; proplasmacytes were observed, and the proportion of proplasmacytes + plasmacytes was 11%.

The patient was finally diagnosed with stage 5 chronic kidney disease, multiple myeloma (light chain lambda, International Staging System [ISS] stage IIIB), and moderate anemia.

Given the patient's fragility, we prescribed dexamethasone combined with thalidomide. Later, a modified regimen of bortezomib + dexamethasone (hereafter referred to as the PD regimen) was given: bortezomib 1.9 mg (1.3 mg/m2) + dexamethasone 20 mg on days 1 and 8 of each month and then only on day 1 of each month because of intolerance. We continued regular hemodialysis with access to a tunneled-cuffed catheter because her vascular conditions were ill-suited for an arteriovenous fistula.

On October 16, 2019, during the hemodialysis procedure, the patient developed dialyzer grade III coagulation, with right lower limb swelling. Vascular Doppler ultrasound revealed deep venous thrombosis of the femoral and popliteal veins of the right lower extremity. An inferior vena cava filter was placed on October 18, 2019, along with low-molecular-weight heparin, urokinase, and warfarin for bridging anticoagulation. After the patient's condition stabilized, the inferior vena cava filter was removed on November 20, 2019.

For anemia, the patient was originally given a subcutaneous injection of 10,000 U of rHuEPO (once a week) at admission. She was also given iron supplementation (ferrous succinate 200 mg, orally, twice a day), and we increased the dosage of erythropoiesis-stimulating agent (ESA), that is, subcutaneous injection of rHuEPO (10,000 U, once a week) + intravenous rHuEPO (3000 U, once a week). Later, the patient developed lower-extremity deep venous thrombosis, which may have been due to multiple myeloma, hyperviscosity, and adverse reactions caused by ESA. Therefore, we temporarily stopped the ESA, and her Hb decreased to 54 g/L. She was given a transfusion of 1 unit of red blood cells on October 22 and 27, 2019. Oral roxadustat was started in December 2019 (100 mg, orally, 3 times/ week) and was gradually adjusted according to the patient's hemoglobin level. The changes in her hemoglobin during treatment are shown in Fig. 5.1.

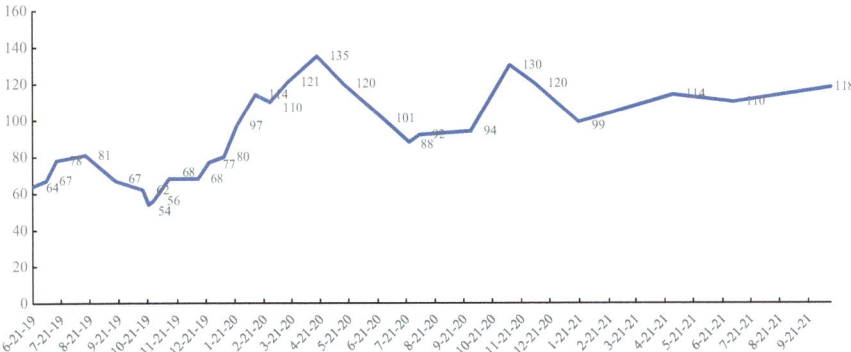

Fig. 5.1 Changes in hemoglobin levels

The patient was followed up for more than 2 years. In September 2021, she received 16 modified PD regimens. The last bone marrow aspirate smear examination (January 2021) revealed a proplasma cell + proplasma cell ratio of 3%, suggesting remission of multiple myeloma, and maintenance hemodialysis treatment was continued (twice a week for 5 hours). The anticoagulant dose was appropriately increased during dialysis; warfarin anticoagulation (1250 μg once a day) was used during dialysis intervals, and the international normalized ratio (INR) was regularly monitored and kept at 2 to 3. The patient had no further thromboembolic events, and hemoglobin concentration was kept at 110 ~ 120 g/L for a long time.

5.2 Discussion

Anemia is a common complication in patients with CKD. The prevalence of anemia in CKD patients in China is 51.5%, while that in patients with CKD stage 5 is up to 90.2% [1]. Anemia is an independent risk factor for cardiovascular complications and affects the prognosis and outcome of CKD patients [2]. In this case, the patient had renal impairment caused by multiple myeloma, and the causes of anemia were multifactorial, including CKD and multiple myeloma. We then created a bortezomib-based treatment plan for patients and adjusted the drug dose and treatment interval according to the patient's tolerance.

In terms of treatment options for renal anemia, the commonly used methods include iron supplementation, ESA, and blood transfusion. ESA is widely used, but it can increase cardiovascular and cerebrovascular events and cause thromboembolism and malignant tumors. In this case, the patient's primary disease was a hematological malignancy, and lower-limb venous thrombosis occurred during treatment; therefore, we needed a better choice for treating her anemia.

Roxadustat, an oral drug for the treatment of renal anemia, can promote erythropoiesis through two key factors, EPO and iron, and improve anemia in CKD patients by stimulating a hypoxic state in humans [3]. Although adverse events such as thromboembolism have also been reported with roxadustat, its incidence of adverse cardiovascular events is not higher than that of ESA [4]. Thus, it is practical for both nondialysis-dependent CKD patients and maintenance hemodialysis patients [5, 6]. In this patient, roxadustat showed excellent efficacy and safety. During follow-up, the dosage of roxadustat was adjusted according to her changes in hemoglobin to keep it stable in the long run and improve her quality of life and prognosis.

References

1. Li Y, Shi H, Wang WM, et al. Prevalence, awareness, and treatment of anemia in Chinese patients with nondialysis chronic kidney disease: first multicenter, cross-sectional study. Medicine. 2016;95(24):e3872.
2. Thavarajah S, Choi MJ. The use of erythropoiesis-stimulating agents in patients with CKD and cancer: a clinical approach. Am J Kidney Dis. 2019;74(5):667–74.
3. Gupta N, Wish JB. Hypoxia-inducible factor prolyl hydroxylase inhibitors: a potential new treatment for anemia in patients with CKD. Am J Kidney Dis. 2017;69(6):815–26.
4. Abdelazeem B, Shehata J, Abbas KS, et al. The efficacy and safety of roxadustat for the treatment of anemia in non-dialysis dependent chronic kidney disease patients: an updated systematic review and meta-analysis of randomized clinical trials. PLoS One. 2022;17(4):e0266243.
5. Chen N, Hao C, Liu BC, et al. Roxadustat treatment for anemia in patients undergoing long-term dialysis. N Engl J Med. 2019;381(11):1011–22.
6. Chen N, Hao C, Peng X, et al. Roxadustat for anemia in patients with kidney disease not receiving dialysis. N Engl J Med. 2019;381(11):1001–10.

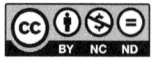

Treatment of a Patient with Peritoneal Dialysis Combined with Erythropoietin-Hyporesponsive Anemia

6

Hong Chu and Jie Dong

6.1 Case Presentation

A 65-year-old woman complained of peritoneal dialysis with renal anemia for 3 years. Three years ago, the patient visited our hospital because of fatigue and vomiting. Her blood pressure was 162/64 mmHg, and laboratory examinations revealed a serum creatinine level of 666.4 μmol/L, a hemoglobin level of 77 g/L, a serum phosphorus level of 1.73 mmol/L, a serum calcium level of 2.32 mmol/L, and an iPTH level of 1061 pg/ml. After comprehensive evaluation, the patient was diagnosed with "chronic kidney disease (CKD) stage 5," and its etiology was considered chronic glomerulonephritis and diabetic nephropathy. The patient was treated with peritoneal dialysis and integrated treatment for CKD, including correction of anemia. She was followed up regularly for 3 years, and no peritoneal dialysis-related acute or chronic complications occurred. The dialysis prescription was adjusted step by step, and the dialysis adequacy urea clearance index (Kt/V) ranged from 1.7 to 2.3. The current dialysis prescription was continuous ambulatory peritoneal dialysis (CAPD) (1.5% peritoneal dialysis solution twice a day and + 2.5% peritoneal dialysis solution twice a day, with 1.9 L of peritoneal dialysis fluid each time, which was stored in the abdomen for 24 hours). At this time, the average ultrafiltration volume was 700 ~ 1000 ml/d, and the average urine volume was 500 ~ 900 ml/d, with a Kt/V of 2.26. The patient's nutritional status was fair, and the albumin concentration was 36 ~ 40 g/L, with no manifestations of volume overload or serious infection. Oral phosphate binders, calcitriol, and cinacalcet were used to treat her CKD mineral and bone metabolism abnormalities (CKD-MBD); the serum phosphorus concentration was 1.73 mmol/L; the calcium concentration was 2.33 mmol/L, and the

H. Chu · J. Dong (✉)
Renal Division, Department of Medicine, Peking University First Hospital,
Peking University Institute of Nephrology, Beijing, China
e-mail: jie.dong@bjmu.edu.cn

© The Author(s) 2025
B.-C. Liu (ed.), *Treatment of Refractory Renal Anemia*,
https://doi.org/10.1007/978-981-97-7636-8_6

27

iPTH concentration was 255.9 pg/ml. The patient was regularly treated with oral iron supplementation and subcutaneous injection of "rHuEPO" for anemia. She exhibited no severe active blood loss and had a serum ferritin concentration of 380 ~ 580 ng/ml and a transferrin saturation of 30% ~ 40% according to regular monitoring. However, her hemoglobin levels continued to be 77 to 85 g/L over the past 6 months, far below the target level.

The patient had a history of chronic glomerulonephritis for 13 years and type 2 diabetes for 12 years. At present, the patient is receiving continuous insulin therapy, and her blood glucose level is well controlled.

Physical examination revealed her blood pressure was 127/53 mmHg; heart rate, 73 bpm; body height, 1.62 m; body weight, 67.2 kg; and body mass index (BMI), 25.61 kg/m^2. The physical examination of the patient's heart, lungs, and abdomen was unremarkable. There was no significant edema in either lower limb. The laboratory examinations of her routine blood tests during rHuEPO treatment are presented in Table 6.1, and hemoglobin concentrations and C-reactive protein (CRP) levels from August 2016 to March 2019 are shown in Figs. 6.1 and 6.2, respectively.

The body fluid volumes from September 2016 to January 2018 during rHuEPO treatment are shown in Table 6.2. Routine stool examination results were negative. Routine blood tests revealed a serum ferritin level of 400.1 μg/L, an iron level of 11.4 μmol/L, a transferrin saturation of 31.5%, a folic acid concentration of >53 nmol/L, and a vitamin B12 concentration of >53 pmol/L. Blood biochemistry examination revealed an albumin level of 36.6 g/L, a creatinine level of 615 μmol/L, a urinary nitrogen level of 16.43 mmol/L, a phosphorus level of 1.73 mmol/L, a calcium level of 2.33 mmol/L, a brain natriuretic peptide level of 160 ng/mL, a CRP level of 2 mg/L, and an iPTH level of 255.9 pg/ml. Thyroid function tests indicated a triiodothyronine level of 1.94 pmol/L, a thyroxine level of 3.9 pmol/L, and a thyroid-stimulating hormone level of 4.84 U/ml. Abdominal ultrasound revealed bilateral renal atrophy, diffuse lesions in both kidneys with multiple cysts, and fatty liver.

A bone marrow smear revealed active bone marrow proliferation with a granulocyte/red blood cell ratio of 1.9:1.0. The cell morphology was approximately normal

Table 6.1 Hematology test results from November 2018 to March 2019

Date	Hb (g/L)	MCV (fl)	MCH (pg)	Ret (109/L)	WBC (109/L)	PLT (109/L)	EPO (10,000 U/week)
Nov. 22, 2018	80	102.1	35.6	90.68	6.19	116	1.0
Dec. 20, 2018	77	104.9	34.9	89.98	6.04	99	1.6
January 24, 2019	77	106.5	35.1	84.20	5.58	128	1.6
February 21, 2019	85	103.7	33.9	123.74	4.93	95	2.0
March 22, 2019	79	103.1	35.3	103.05	7.37	150	2.0

Note: *Hb* hemoglobin; *MCV* mean corpuscular volume; *MCH* mean corpuscular hemoglobin; *Ret* reticulocyte count; *WBC* white blood cell count; *PLT* platelet count; *EPO* erythropoietin

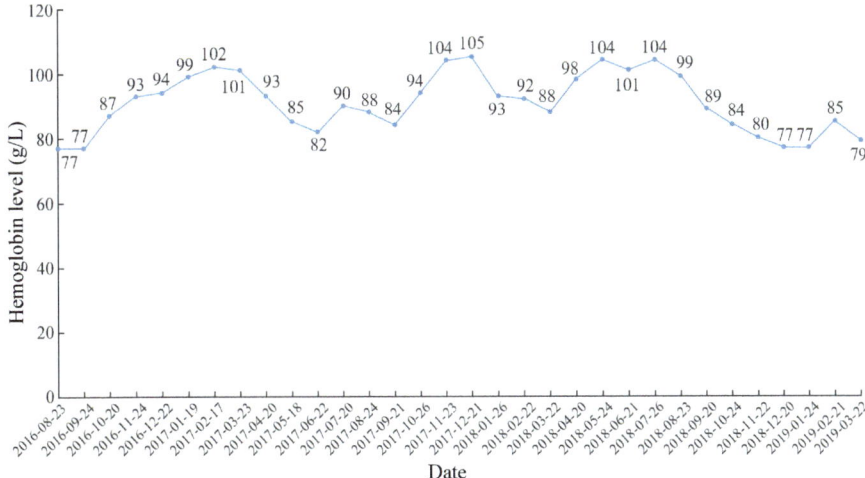

Fig. 6.1 Hemoglobin concentrations during rHuEPO treatment. Note: *rHuEPO* recombinant human erythropoietin; subcutaneous rHuEPO 9000 U/week from Aug 23, 2016 to Apr 19, 2017; 10,000 U/week from Apr 20, 2017 to Aug 23, 2017; 15,000 U/week from Aug 24, 2017 to Sep 20, 2017; 16,000 U/week from Sep 21, 2017 to Oct 26, 2017

From October 26 to June 20, 2018, the rHuEPO dose was 17,500 U/week; from June 21 to December 19, 2018, the rHuEPO dose was 10,000 U/week; from December 20, 2018, to February 20, 2019, the rHuEPO dose was 16,000 U/week; and from February 21 to March 22, 2019, the rHuEPO dose was 20,000 U/week

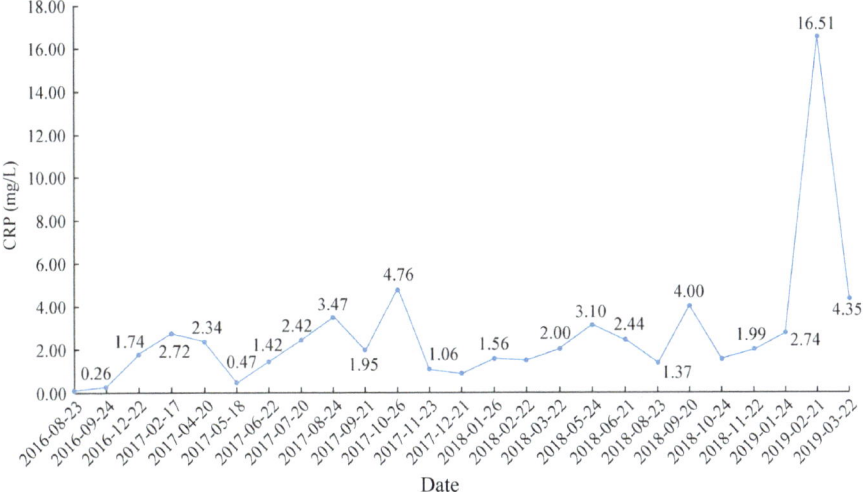

Fig. 6.2 Changes in C-reactive protein. Note: *CRP* C-reactive protein

Table 6.2 Patient volume profile

Date	Extracellular fluid/total body fluid (E/T)	Volume overload/extracellular fluid (OH/E)
September 27, 2016	0.480	0.119
October 25, 2016	0.473	0.061
January 24, 2017	0.469	0.028
March 28, 2017	0.465	0.073
October 31, 2017	0.478	0.084
January 30, 2018	0.480	0.042

Note: *E* extracellular fluid; *OH* volume overload; *T* total body fluid volume

at all stages of the granulocytic lineage. In the red blood cell population, the erythroblasts had large cell bodies, and the mature red blood cells varied in size and were arranged in a rouleaux pattern. Lymphocytes accounted for 5% of the cells; monocytes accounted for 3% of the cells, and plasma cells accounted for 2% of the cells. There were 14 megakaryocytes, and no plate-producing megakaryocytes were observed. Extracellular iron (+ + + +) and intracellular iron 32/50 (type I, 20; type II, 9; and type III, 3) were detected. Flow cytometry revealed mildly abnormal development of granulocytic cells, and the proportion of granulocytic blasts was not high. Genetic testing did not reveal leukemia- or myelodysplastic syndrome (MDS)-related genes.

Main Clinical Diagnoses
1. Stage 5 chronic kidney disease (continuous ambulatory peritoneal dialysis)
2. Renal hypertension
3. Renal anemia
4. Mineral metabolism disorders
5. Secondary hyperparathyroidism
6. Type 2 diabetes mellitus and diabetic nephropathy
7. Chronic glomerulonephritis

6.2   Clinical Treatment Process

Phase I (December 20, 2018 to August 27, 2019)

1. The treatment plan was as follows:
    1. Exclusion of current infections, such as infections of the eyes, ears, nose, and throat, oral cavity, infective endocarditis, and obstetrics and gynecology.

2. Continued oral iron supplementation to maintain ferritin and transferrin saturation.

3. Replacement of rHuEPO (10,000 U, twice a week, subcutaneous injection) with rHuEPO-β (5,000 U, twice a week, subcutaneous injection) and a gradual increase in the dose to 5000 U three times a week according to the hemoglobin level.

2. Therapeutic effect: After the application of rHuEPO-β, the hemoglobin level stabilized at 90 g/L. Reticulocyte (Ret) levels were not significantly increased (Fig. 6.3), and iron utilization was not significantly improved (Table 6.3).

Phase II (August 28, 2019 to July 15, 2021)

1. Treatment prescription: The administration of rHuEPO-β was stopped, and the patient was given oral HIF-PHI120 mg three times a week.

2. Therapeutic effect: The hemoglobin levels increased significantly; the reticulocyte levels increased (Fig. 6.3), and the iron utilization improved; iron-related parameter levels and C-reactive protein levels are listed in Table 6.3. The patient was still treated with HIF-PHI at a dosage of 100 to 120 mg three times a week, and the hemoglobin concentrations ranged from 100 to 120 g/L (Fig. 6.4), without significant associated adverse effects.

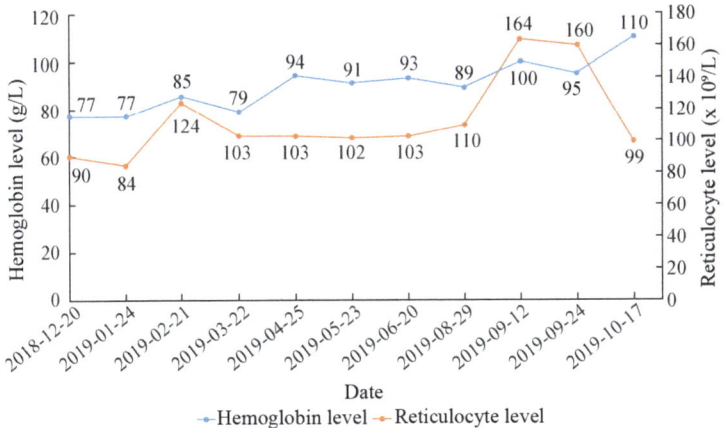

Fig. 6.3 Hemoglobin and reticulocyte changes. Note: From December 20, 2018 to February 20, 2019, rHuEPO 3 times/week, 10,000 U, 3000 U, and 3000 U, respectively; from February 21 to April 24, 2019, rHuEPO 10,000 U 2 times/week; from April 25 to June 19, 2019, application of RHuEPO-β 5000 U, bid; from June 20 to August 27, 2019, rHuEPO-β 5000 U, tid; from August 28 to October 17, 2019, roxadustat 120 mg, tid

Table 6.3 Iron status and C-reactive protein monitoring

Date	January 24, 2019	February 21, 2019	April 25, 2019	July 25, 2019	October 17, 2019
Total iron-binding capacity (μmol/L)	37.8	34.0	36.2	32.7	38.7
Ferritin (μg/L)	387.9	580.3	400.1	460.6	432.7
Serum iron (μmol/L)	12.7	13.7	11.4	12.0	18.3
Transferrin saturation (%)	33.6	40.3	31.5	36.7	47.3
C-reactive protein (mg/L)	2.7	16.5	2.0	4.7	5.7

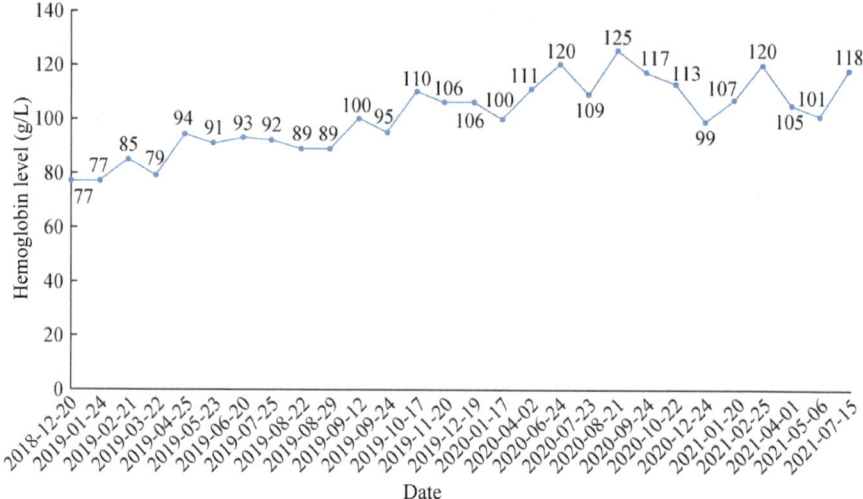

Fig. 6.4 Hemoglobin follow-up results. Note: From December 20, 2018 to February 20, 2019, the patient was administered rHuEPO 3 times/week, 10,000 U, 3000 U, or 3000 U; from February 21 to April 24, 2019, the patient was administered rHuEPO10000U, 2 times/week; from April 25 to June 2019

On July 19, 2019, the patient was treated with rHuEPO-β 5000 U twice a week; from June 20 to April 27, 2019, the patient was treated with rHuEPO-β 5000 U three times a week; from August 28, 2019 to August 20, 2020, the patient was treated with roxadustat 120 mg three times a week; from August 21 to December 23, 2020, the patient was treated with roxadustat 100 mg three times a week; from December 24, 2020 to February 24, 2021, the patient was treated with roxadustat 120 mg three times a week; and from February 25, 2021 to July 15, 2021, the patient was treated with roxadustat three times a week (100 mg, 120 mg each time)

6.3   Discussion

The patient was an elderly woman who was diagnosed with CKD stage 5, chronic glomerulonephritis, and diabetic nephropathy. She was given CAPD and CKD integrated treatment. rHuEPO and iron were administered to correct her anemia; however, the efficacy of these treatments for anemia remained poor.

1. Analysis of the anemia characteristics

According to the results of the routine blood examination (Table 6.1), the patient's hemoglobin level continued to be low, indicating normocytic normochromic anemia. Ret levels were not significantly increased, and the WBC and PLT counts were normal.

After reviewing the hemoglobin and rHuEPO therapeutic plan (Fig. 6.1), the patient had been treated with regular subcutaneous rHuEPO for anemia for 3 years, especially in the past 6 months, and the dose of rHuEPO was continuously increased to maintain hemoglobin stability. The subcutaneous dose of PO reached 300 U/kg per week, but her hemoglobin levels continued to be substandard. Therefore, ESA hyporesponsiveness was considered.

2. Causes of ESA hyporesponsiveness

After anemia caused by bleeding, hemolysis, solid tumors, hematological malignancies, or the use of special drugs was excluded, the following six factors were considered.

2.1. Hematopoietic raw material deficiency: Iron deficiency is the most common cause of hyporesponsiveness to ESAs; however, this patient had been regularly treated with oral iron. Her serum ferritin concentration ranged from 380 to 580 µg/L, and her transferrin saturation ranged from 30% to 40%. This patient had no evidence of folate or vitamin B12 deficiency.

2.2. Inflammatory disease: The IgM test for human parvovirus B19 was negative, and there was no evidence of hepatitis B or C infection. No other evidence of infection was found. However, considering that the CRP concentration was between 2.0 and 16.5 mg/L, the presence of occult infection or a chronic inflammatory state could not be excluded.

2.3. Hyperparathyroidism: The patient was regularly treated with oral phosphate binders, calcitriol, and cinacalcet for CKD-MBD and currently has a serum phosphorus concentration of 1.73 mmol/L, a serum calcium concentration of 2.33 mmol/L, and an iPTH concentration of 255.9 pg/mL. In the past 6 months, her iPTH concentration had ranged from 200 to 300 pg/mL; therefore, there was no evidence of severe hyperparathyroidism.

2.4. Inadequate dialysis: The patient underwent peritoneal dialysis and regular follow-up, and her treatment compliance was good. No acute or chronic complications related to peritoneal dialysis occurred. The dialysis adequacy met the Kt/V 1.7–2.3 standard.

2.5. Volume loading: Volume load is one of the reasons for the hyporesponsiveness of peritoneal dialysis patients to rHuEPO treatment, but no severe volume overload occurred in this patient during peritoneal dialysis treatment. BNP was monitored and measured in the range of 100 ~ 300 ng/ml and combined with the results of the bioelectrical impedance assessment; the volume load was not significantly correlated with hemoglobin fluctuations (Table 6.2).

2.6. rHuEPO antibody-mediated pure red cell aplasia or other hematologic disorders: Based on the results of bone marrow aspiration, relevant diseases were excluded.

In summary, the patient had ESA hyporesponsiveness, which may be associated with impaired iron utilization, occult infection, or a state of chronic inflammation.

Therefore, the treatment plan was adjusted into three main aspects: (1) continue oral iron; (2) replace rHuEPO with rHuE-PO-β, noting that the efficacy is poor; and (3) further suspend rHuEPO-β and change to oral HIF-PHI treatment. During follow-up, the patient's hemoglobin concentration increased significantly; her iron utilization improved, and in the next 2 years of follow-up, her hemoglobin concentration basically reached the standard, and her anemia significantly improved.

6.4   Conclusion

This is an elderly female patient on peritoneal dialysis with ESA hyporesponsiveness. The patient's anemia was successfully improved after switching to HIF-PHI. It is important to give the patient regular detection of hemoglobulin and iron status for anemia management by monitoring the efficacy of the drugs [1]. The long-term use of ESA therapy may produce ESA hyporesponsiveness in some patients, and this hyporesponsiveness may be related to CKD-related inflammatory responses and the oxidative stress status. Chronic inflammation can aggravate anemia through a variety of mechanisms, which mainly include inhibition of bone marrow erythroid system proliferation, increased erythrocyte phagocytosis, inhibition of EPO production, increased hepatic secretion of hepcidin, and iron utilization disorders [2–4].

Anemia status is closely related to the prognosis of patients with end-stage renal disease, and improving anemia has important clinical value. The Dialysis Outcomes and Practice Patterns Study (DOPPS) of 4000 hemodialysis patients revealed that for every 10 g/L increase in hemoglobin, the mortality rate decreased by 5% [5]. HIF-PHI mimics the physiological process of EPO production and iron utilization by stabilizing HIF to regulate downstream genes. This results in the upregulation of EPO, the EPO receptor, and hepcidin-related genes and proteins under hypoxic conditions, thereby improving renal anemia [6, 7]. Chen et al. (2019) reported that in a phase III clinical trial of long-term dialysis patients, the hemoglobin level and HIF-PHI therapeutic dose were similar to that in the HIF-PHI treatment group, the subgroup with elevated CRP, and the subgroup with normal CRP. However, in the rHuEPO treatment group, although the rHuEPO dose required for the treatment of the subgroup with elevated CRP was higher, the hemoglobin level was lower. These findings suggest that HIF-PHI therapy maintains a relatively stable hemoglobin level without causing inflammation; thus, it is speculated that these drugs can partially improve ESA hyporesponsiveness [8].

References

1. Chinese Society of Nephrology Consensus Expert Group on the Diagnosis and Treatment of Renal Anemia. Chinese expert consensus on diagnosis and treatment of renal anemia (2018 revision). Chin J Nephrol. 2018;34:860–6.
2. Bradbury BD, Critchlow CW, Weir MR, Ron S, Mahesh K, Hakim RH. Impact of elevated C-reactive protein levels on erythropoiesis-stimulating agent (ESA) dose and responsiveness in hemodialysis patients. Nephrol Dial Transplant. 2009;24:919–25.
3. Locatelli F, Simeone A, Bruno M, Camilla M, Lucia DV, Stefano A, Walter DS, Antonella M, Giuliano B, Marcello A, Bruno C, Carmine Z. Nutritional-inflammation status and resistance to erythropoietin therapy in haemodialysis patients. Nephrol Dial Transplant. 2006;21:991–8.
4. Zarychanski R, Houston DS. Anemia of chronic disease: a harmful disorder or an adaptive, beneficial response? CMAJ. 2008;179:333–7.
5. Locatelli F, Pisoni RL, Christian C, Juergen B, Andreucci VE, Luis P, Roger G, Feldman HI, Port FK, Held PJ. Anaemia in haemodialysis patients of five European countries: Association with morbidity and mortality in the Dialysis Outcomes and Practice Patterns Study (DOPPS). Nephrol Dial Transplant. 2004;19:121–32.
6. Fu Y, Yan T, Bicheng L. Research progress of hypoxia-inducible factor-proline hydroxylase inhibitor in the treatment of renal anemia. Chin J Nephrol. 2020;36:726–30.
7. Kaplan JM, Neeraj S, Sean D. Hypoxia-inducible factor and its role in the management of anemia in chronic kidney disease. Int J Mol Sci. 2018;19:389.
8. Chen N, Chuanming H, Bi-Cheng L, Hongli L, Caili W, Changying X, Xinling L, Gengru J, Zhengrong L, Xuemei L, Li Z, Laimin L, Jianqin W, Ming-Hui Z, Zhihong L, Guang-Yan C, Li H, Robert L, Chunrong W, Cameron L, Thomas N, Lynda S, Yu K-HP. Roxadustat treatment for anemia in patients undergoing long-term dialysis. N Engl J Med. 2019;381:1011–22.

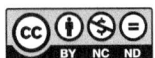

Treatment of Renal Anemia with Hyporesponsive to ESA Due to Unknown Inflammatory Status Reason

7

Mo Zhang and Yinke Du

7.1 Case Presentation

A 44-year-old female patient was admitted to the renal department of our hospital 4 years ago due to "fatigue and proteinuria." Since the onset of the disease, she presented with eyelid and lower limb edema and no nocturia with approximately 1500 mL/24H of urine volume. Routine urine examination indicated 3+ urine protein and negative urine occult blood. Moreover, blood urea nitrogen (BUN) was 10.8 mmol/L; serum creatinine (Scr) was 106 μmol/L; albumin was 31.2 g/L; serum calcium was 1.98 mmol/L; serum phosphorus was 1.56 mmol/L; hemoglobin was 102 g/L; white blood cell count was 6.56×10^9/L; and platelet count was 215×10^9/L. Tumor biomarkers, serum protein electrophoresis, immunoglobulin, rheumatism indicators, and hepatitis parameters were all negative. Renal biopsy diagnosed diabetic nephropathy. The patient had a 12-year history of diabetes with hypertension. The patient received pharmacotherapy for glycemic control; antihypert, ertensive regimen included valsartan and benidipine. Additionally, weekly subcutaneous injections of recombinant human erythropoietin (6000–9000 U) combined with oral iron polysaccharide complex were administered to ameliorate renal anemia, while calcium acetate was utilized to correct chronic kidney disease-mineral and bone disorder (CKD-MBD). Furthermore, a low-protein diet was implemented alongside traditional Chinese medicine (TCM) preparations to decelerate the progression of renal function. Blood pressure and blood sugar control were deemed satisfactory, and lower limb edema disappeared.

Over the following 2 years, her hemoglobin was maintained at 85–105 g/L, ferritin at 121–286 μg/L, and transferrin saturation at 15%–36%. Two years ago, the re-examination of renal function tests showed that blood urea nitrogen (BUN) was 22.4–24.8 mmol/L, and serum creatinine (Scr) was 844–1076 μmol/L. At the

M. Zhang · Y. Du (✉)
The First Hospital of China Medical University, Shenyang, China

© The Author(s) 2025
B.-C. Liu (ed.), *Treatment of Refractory Renal Anemia*,
https://doi.org/10.1007/978-981-97-7636-8_7

same time, blood pressure was difficult to control, reaching up to 210/110 mmHg. She experienced shortness of breath, difficulty lying down at night, severe lower limb edema, and reduced urine volume, approximately 500 mL/24H. Her BNP was 4120 pg/mL, and troponin was 0.03 ug/L. Grade IV left heart dysfunction was diagnosed, and maintenance hemodialysis was initiated at the blood purification center of our hospital thrice a week for 4 hours each time. After 2 weeks of hemodialysis, both lower limb edema and dyspnea improved, and BNP was re-examined at 820 pg/mL. Simultaneously, blood routine examination showed the following results: white blood cell count, 6.88 × 1012/L; hemoglobin, 86 g/L; platelet count, 273 × 109/L; proportion of neutrophils, 68.7%; ferritin, 221 µg/L; transferrin saturation, 21.4%; Blood electrolytes: potassium, 3.98 mmol/L; calcium, 2.12 mmol/L; inorganic phosphorus, 2.5 mmol /L; serum bicarbonate, 22.1 mmol/L; parathyroid hormone, 63.82 pmol/L; fecal occult blood test, negative; PCT, 0.23ug/L; folic acid, 4 ng/mL; vitamin B12, 488 pg/mL; albumin, 41 g/L; CRP, 36 mg/L; and CD4, 146/UL, Lung CT showed no infection. For the correction of renal anemia, recombinant human erythropoietin 12000 u was administered per week. During the treatment process, factors such as infection, active bleeding, iron deficiency, and malnutrition have been excluded. Moreover, anemia is currently considered in patients with microinflammatory status, so we have changed the treatment regimen: EPO was changed to roxadustat 100 mg orally three times a week. Three months later, her hemoglobin increased to 102 g/L, and it has been maintained at 106–121 g/L for nearly a year. CRP tests range from 18 to 45 mg/L. Changes in hemoglobin levels during treatment are shown in Fig. 7.1. Changes in ferritin and transferrin saturation during treatment are shown in Fig. 7.2.

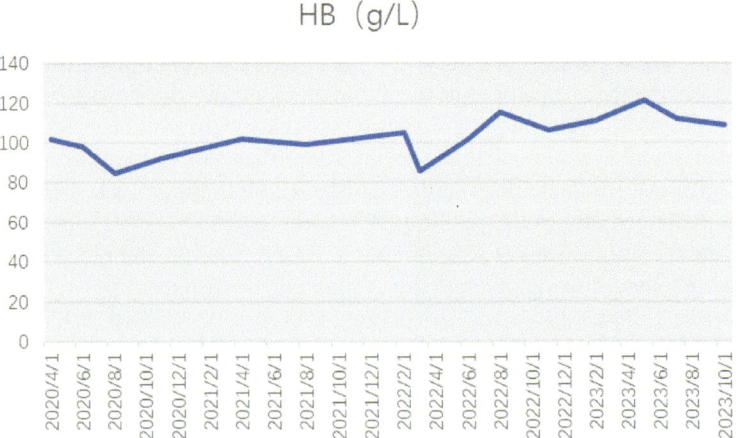

Fig. 7.1 Hemoglobin changes in the patient

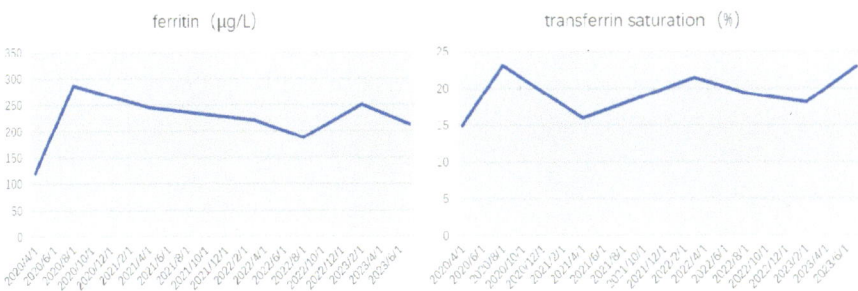

Fig. 7.2 Changes in ferritin and transferrin saturation during treatment

7.2 Discussion

Microinflammatory status is one of the important conditions complicated in hemodialysis, which can significantly affect the patient's response to rHuEPO when it is used for renal anemia. The possible reasons for this phenomenon may be the following: (1) The proinflammatory factors in the body act on different stages of erythropoiesis, inhibit erythropoiesis, reduce the sensitivity of the body to erythropoietin, and inhibit the synthesis of endogenous erythropoietin. (2) The increase of hemoferritin in the inflammatory response prevents the release of iron to the precursors of red blood cells, inhibits the absorption of iron by the body, and leads to iron utilization disorders and physiological iron deficiency. At present, serum ferritin is commonly used in clinical practice to reflect the iron storage in the body. Because it is an acute reaction product, it will also increase in inflammation, tumor, and other conditions; thus, the iron status of the body cannot be accurately evaluated, resulting in iatrogenic iron deficiency. (3) Inflammatory signals activate macrophages, accelerate the clearance of red blood cells, shorten the life of red blood cells, and decrease hemoglobin. (4) Upregulation of hepcidin inhibits iron absorption: Increased hepcidin levels in MHD patients may be related to decreased hepcidin excretion, functional iron deficiency, anemia, and microinflammation caused by decreased renal function. Elevated levels of hepcidin block iron release from macrophages and jejunal cells, which causes insufficient iron transport in the erythroid bone marrow, resulting in iron-deficient erythropoiesis and ultimately functional or relative iron deficiency [1, 2].

Microinflammatory states are more common in patients treated with dialysis, but different levels of microinflammatory states have different responses to the treatment of renal anemia with rHuEPO, that is, the higher the level of microinflammatory factors, the worse the treatment effect of anemia. In clinical treatment, monitoring the level of microinflammatory factors in patients treated with dialysis, adjusting the dosage of EPO, and giving appropriate anti-inflammatory intervention are the new targets for the treatment of renal anemia. In a micro-inflammatory state, the dosage of EPO and iron can be appropriately increased, but the dosage should not be excessive. Peter Bdrdny found that the low erythropoietin reactivity caused by microinflammation can be basically corrected by increasing the therapeutic dose of rHuEPO. However, excessive dose of rHuEPO will cause the level of hemoglobu-1 in (Hb) to increase too fast or too high, increasing the risk of related adverse reactions. At the same time, it does not have a good cost-benefit ratio.

Roxadustat, as a representative of HIF-PHI, is capable of regulating erythropoiesis comprehensively, correcting anemia, and enhancing hemoglobin levels via multiple steps, and its efficacy remains unaffected by microinflammatory conditions [3]. Roxadustat regulated the levels of inflammatory factors, increased iron utilization, and altered the diversity and abundance of the gut microbiota, especially in terms of SCFA-producing bacteria, thus alleviating ESA resistance [4]. Research has demonstrated that roxadustat could effectively attenuate the influence of microinflammatory state to anemia correction. Possible reasons may be related with its unique mechanism by stimulating the endogenous production of EPO and restoring the disturbed iron metabolism.

References

1. Kalantar Zadeh K, McAllister CJ, Lehn RS, et al. Effect of malnutrition inflammation complex syndrome on EPO hypo—responsiveness in maintenance hemodialysis patients. Am J Kidney Dis. 2003;42(4):761—773.
2. Martone M, Zanchi R, Panzetta G, et al. Role of iron deficiency in erythropoietin sensitivity in dialysis patients with elevated C reactive protein. G Ital Nefrol. 2003;20(1):31–7.
3. Santos-Silva A, Ribeiro S, Reis F, et al. Hepcidin in chronic kidney disease anemia. Vitam Horm. 2019;110:243–64.
4. Santos EJF, Dias RSC, Lima JFDB, et al. Erythropoietin resistance in patients with chronic kidney disease: current perspectives. Int J Nephrol Renovasc Dis. 2020;13:231–7.

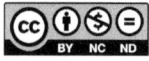

Part II

CKD Anemia with Inflammation or Infection

Infection is a common and serious complication in patients with chronic kidney disease, especially those receiving peritoneal dialysis or hemodialysis. Infection can easily exacerbate anemia symptoms in kidney patients and lead to a poor response to ESA treatment. Owing to systemic inflammatory responses, these patients have increased levels of hepcidin and iron utilization disorders, which manifest as hyper-ferritinemia or functional iron deficiency. Infection or inflammatory responses are important reasons for the low treatment target rate of renal anemia in dialysis patients in China. Anti-infection or control of inflammation is the basic strategy for treating such patients, but how to effectively improve anemia in patients is still a challenge faced by clinicians. In previous clinical trials related to the application of ESAs and roxadustat for the treatment of renal anemia, patients with infection or obvious inflammation were excluded from the trials. Therefore, currently there is a lack of evidence-based medical evidence to guide the treatment of such patients. In this part, we present several experiences in the use of roxadustat to treat renal anemia complicated by infection, with the aim of providing valuable references and inspiration for the treatment of such complex clinical cases.

Anemia Treatment with Roxadustat in a Peritoneal Dialysis Patient During Omicron Virus Infection: A Case Report

8

Qinghua Yang, Jiaxiang Ding, and Feng Yu

8.1   Case Presentation

A 78-year-old male was admitted due to fever, cough, and fatigue for 1 week. The patient was diagnosed with diabetes more than 30 years ago and had poor control of blood glucose levels with oral drugs. Five years prior to admission, the patient had proteinuria and mildly elevated serum creatinine and was diagnosed with diabetic nephropathy. More than 1 year prior to admission, his creatinine level increased to 486 μmol/L, and his hemoglobin level was 83 g/L; these levels were accompanied by fatigue, wheezing, elevated blood pressure, anemia, and a urine volume of 1000 mL/day. The patient was diagnosed with "end-stage renal disease." The patient underwent peritoneal dialysis catheterization and peritoneal dialysis 1 year prior to admission.

For the treatment of anemia, the hemoglobin (Hb) level was regularly measured monthly. Roxadustat 50 mg three times a week and polysaccharide-iron composite capsules 150 mg per day were taken. The Hb concentration reached 127 g/L after 1 month. Roxadustat was reduced to 50 mg twice per week. The Hb concentration was maintained between 120 and 130 g/L. One week prior, the patient was admitted due to Omicron virus infection and developed anorexia and diarrhea. He lost 2 kilograms of weight in 1 month and exhibited fatigue and dysuria.

Examination at admission revealed a temperature of 36.6 °C, pulse of 62 beats/minute, respiration rate of 19 breaths/minute, blood pressure of 104/59 mmHg, weight of 49.2 kg, anemic appearance, and no enlargement of systemic superficial lymph nodes. The breath sounds in both lungs were coarse, without dry or moist rales. The left heart border was enlarged; the heart rate was 62 beats/minute; the heart rhythm was regular, and no pathological murmur was heard. The abdomen

Q. Yang · J. Ding (✉) · F. Yu
Renal Division, Peking University International Hospital, Beijing, China
e-mail: dingjiaxiang@pkuih.edu.cn

© The Author(s) 2025
B.-C. Liu (ed.), *Treatment of Refractory Renal Anemia*,
https://doi.org/10.1007/978-981-97-7636-8_8

43

was soft and nontender. The peritoneal dialysis catheter was fixed in place, and no edema in either lower limb was observed.

Past medical history: Hypertension for more than 20 years and coronary heart disease for more than 1 year. Diabetic fundus lesions were treated surgically.

Diagnosis on admission: Omicron virus infection (mild type); diabetic nephropathy, chronic kidney disease stage 5D (peritoneal dialysis), renal anemia, and renal hypertension; coronary atherosclerotic heart disease and cardiac function grade II (New York Heart Association [NYHA] class); and hypertension.

Treatment course: The patient had a good response to roxadustat in the past, and anemia worsened after drug withdrawal. After oral administration of the drug resumed, the patient's anemia resolved, but anemia occurred again after the recent Omicron virus infection. Relevant examinations after admission revealed positive results for Omicron virus nucleic acid and negative results for coronavirus antibodies. Routine blood tests indicated that the leukocyte count was 5.48×10^9/L, Hb was 104 g/L, serum ferritin was 371.2 μ/L, serum iron was 16.6 μmol/L (reference range, 10–36.7), transferrin was 1740 mg/L (reference range, 170–340), total iron-binding capacity was 38.2 μmol/L (reference range, 50–77), transferrin saturation was 43.5%, vitamin B12 was >1476 pmol/L, and folic acid was 26.08 nmol/L. Stool occult blood test showed negative. Biochemistry panel test revealed that serum creatinine was 514 μmol/L, urea was 15.76 mmol/L, blood calcium was 2.25 mmol/L, blood phosphorus was 1.47 mmol/L, albumin was 17.5 g/L, and parathyroid hormone was 43.8 ng/L. The high-sensitivity C-reactive protein concentration was 48.55 mg/L (reference range, 0–3), and N-terminal pro b-type natriuretic peptide was 3806 pg/mL (reference range, < 125).

Chest computed tomography scan revealed scattered infectious lesions in both lungs. Cardiac ultrasound revealed left ventricular hypertrophy, aortic valve calcification with mild regurgitation, mild mitral and tricuspid regurgitation, a widened ascending aorta, and a 63% reduction in diastolic function and left ventricular ejection fraction. Considering that the patient had an Omicron virus infection, the patient was given 100 mg of tritiated Remdesivir hydrobromide tablets daily for 3 days.

The patient's case was characterized by anemia, a fair therapeutic effect of roxadustat, Omicron virus infection, mildly decreased hemoglobin, increased ferritin, normal transferrin saturation, and severe hypoalbuminemia. After admission to correct hypoproteinemia, peritoneal dialysis machine therapy was performed. Due to anemia, 70 mg roxadustat was given three times a week. Two weeks later, the level of C-reactive protein decreased to 4.62 mg/L, and the level of hemoglobin increased to 109 g/L (Fig. 8.1). His cough and fatigue also disappeared.

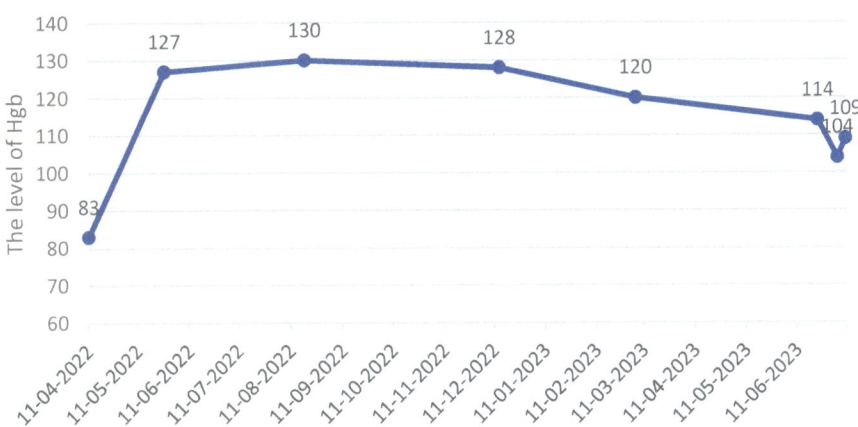

Fig. 8.1 Changes in hemoglobin levels

8.2   Discussion

The clinical features of this case were as follows: elderly patients with an acute course, previously correctable renal anemia, and a recent decrease in hemoglobin and increase in serum ferritin due to infection with a new severe acute respiratory syndrome coronavirus 2 (SARS-CoV-2) variant, i.e., Omicron. An inflammatory state was present. Once the diagnosis of renal anemia is made, the etiology of anemia can be investigated. Common causes of anemia include iron deficiency, chronic blood loss, inflammatory conditions, hyperparathyroidism, and inadequate dialysis [1]. Relevant examinations were performed after admission, and the patient had no absolute or relative iron deficiency. Serum ferritin was increased in this patient; ferritin is not only an indicator of iron storage but also an acute reactive protein that is significantly increased in patients with inflammation or tumors. Ferritin is noted to increase in patients with iron metabolism disorders, and low serum iron is a feature of chronic inflammatory anemia [2]. On the basis of the patient's infection with a new coronavirus variant, inflammatory state, and gastrointestinal symptoms, which affected eating and caused hypoproteinemia, the patient received enhanced nutrition supplementation and antiviral treatment to improve the inflammatory state and correct the cause of anemia.

In this case, chronic inflammation, anemia, and severe hypoproteinemia interacted with each other. The resulting inflammatory state was associated with hemodynamic changes, oxidative stress, intestinal microcirculation, and barrier dysfunction, leading to endotoxin leakage into the blood and activation of the neurohormonal system [3]. Notably, the peritoneal dialysate itself weakens the microcirculation and barrier function of the intestine and is more likely to lead to increased endotoxin. Therefore, gastrointestinal symptoms may be related to the inflammatory state of patients. The mechanism of anemia due to chronic inflammation is currently thought to involve hepcidin, as it causes changes in iron metabolism, including reduced iron absorption in the gastrointestinal tract and iron phagocytosis by macrophages. Therefore, anemia can be exacerbated in dialysis patients under inflammatory conditions [4].

Roxadustat can improve anemia in dialysis patients with inflammatory conditions [5]. Compared with conventional erythropoietin (EPO) therapy, roxadustat therapy can improve iron metabolism [6]. Previous studies have demonstrated that roxadustat downregulates hepcidin expression at the gene transcription level and upregulates the expression of duodenal cytochrome B, the divalent metal ion transporter, and transferrin and its receptor. Ultimately, the result of the alterations in iron metabolism is increased absorption of iron in the gastrointestinal tract, which promotes iron transport to bone marrow for hematopoiesis [7]. Previous clinical studies have confirmed the ability of roxadustat to downregulate hepcidin expression and correct anemia even in patients with iron deficiency [6]. In this case, roxadustat was found to be effective in correcting anemia after dialysis. Due to infection with the novel coronavirus variant, the Hb level decreased slightly but then recovered during roxadustat treatment. Roxadustat can prevent large fluctuations in hemoglobin during SARS-CoV-2 infection.

It is important to analyze the cause of worsening anemia in dialysis patients. Additionally, we need to deepen our understanding of the mechanisms of action of roxadustat in correcting anemia and its advantages. Roxadustat can be used to treat anemia in dialysis patients with Omicron virus infection.

References

1. Anon. Chinese expert consensus on diagnosis and treatment of renal anemia. Chin J Nephrol. 2018;34(11):860–6.
2. Zhang M, Wang X. Diagnosis and treatment of inflammatory anemia. J Clin Hematol. 2019;32(1):68–71.
3. Dick SA, Epelman S. Chronic heart failure and inflammation: what do we really know? Circ Res. 2016;119(1):159–76.
4. Camaschella C. Iron and hepcidin: a story of recycling and balance. Hematology Am Soc Hematol Educ Program. 2013;2013:1–8.
5. Chen N, Hao C, Liu BC, et al. Roxadustat treatment for anemia in patients undergoing long-term dialysis. N Engl J Med. 2019;381(11):1011–22.
6. Besarab A, Chernyavskaya E, Motylev I, et al. Roxadustat (FG-4592): correction of anemia in incident dialysis patients. J Am Soc Nephrol. 2016;27(4):1225–33.
7. Li ZL, Tu Y, Liu BC. Treatment of renal anemia with roxadustat: advantages and achievement. Kidney Dis (Basel). 2020;6(2):65–73.

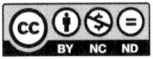

Use of a Hypoxia-Inducible Factor Prolyl Hydroxylase Inhibitor in a Peritoneal Dialysis Patient with Coronavirus Disease 2019

9

Minxia Li, Yuehong Li, Wei Wang, and Zhen Zhuang

9.1 Case Presentation

A 70-year-old male on peritoneal dialysis presented with a 3-day history of fever. He was hospitalized for hyperpyrexia, cough, expectoration, asthenia, and worsening dyspnea, and he was diagnosed with coronavirus disease 2019 (COVID-19) pneumonia by nucleic acid testing. He had a 30-year history of hypertension and hyperlipidemia and had been treated with an angiotensin II receptor blocker, calcium channel blocker (CCB), and statin for 30 years. He had a 17-year history of glomerular nephritis. His serum creatinine gradually increased over 10 years. Finally, he started treatment with continuous ambulatory peritoneal dialysis (CAPD) 2 years prior to admission and was followed up regularly at our peritoneal dialysis center. The CAPD program consisted of 3 exchanges/day with peritoneal dialysate solution (Fresenius AG, 1.5–2.5% glucose, 2.5% × 2000 mL long-term storage at night). His daily ultrafiltration volume was approximately 1000 mL, and his urine volume was 400–500 mL/day. The patient was started on recombinant human erythropoietin (rh-EPO) at a dosage of 3000 U twice a week for anemia treatment 3 years prior to admission. Hemoglobin levels remained between 107 and 120 g/L.

Physical examination revealed a blood pressure of 122/78 mmHg，temperature 39.6 °C, pulse rate 102 bpm, respiratory rate 30 breaths/minute, and body weight 74 kg. The oxygen saturation is 80% without supplemental oxygen which is going up to 90% with oxygen therapy. There is no rash, edema, lymphadenopathy, or organomegaly.

Laboratory tests revealed the following results: white blood cell (WBC) count, 9.27×10^9/L; red blood cell (RBC) count, 2.88×10^{12}/L; hemoglobin level, 84 g/L; platelet count, 131×10^9/L; lymphocyte count, 0.41×10^9/L; neutrophil count,

M. Li · Y. Li (✉) · W. Wang · Z. Zhuang
Beijing Tsinghua Changgung Hospital, School of Clinical Medicine, Tsinghua University, Beijing, China
e-mail: LMXA01104@btch.edu.cn; LYHA01051@btch.edu.cn

© The Author(s) 2025
B.-C. Liu (ed.), *Treatment of Refractory Renal Anemia*,
https://doi.org/10.1007/978-981-97-7636-8_9

8.51 × 109/L; neutrophil percentage, 91.8%; C-reactive protein (CRP), 224.1 mg/L; blood urea nitrogen, 24.9 mmol/L; creatinine, 1184 µmol/L; uric acid, 338 µmol/L; serum total protein, 78.3 g/L; albumin, 36.2 g/L; serum calcium, 2.34 mmol/L; and phosphorus, 1.77 mmol/L. The patient's intact parathyroid hormone (iPTH) level was 198 ng/L. Serological test results for tumor markers and anti-nuclear and anti-double-stranded DNA were all negative. He was negative for other respiratory viruses, hepatitis B, hepatitis C, and HIV. Serum protein electrophoresis and Coombs test results were negative. There was no evidence of gastrointestinal bleeding (the fecal occult blood test was negative). The levels of biomarkers of iron storage and function were as follows: iron, 14.6 µmol/L; transferrin saturation, 16.8%; and ferritin, 641.7 µg/L. Chest computed tomography revealed bilateral multilobular patchy and ground-glass opacities indicating pneumonia, bilateral interstitial inflammation, and bilateral emphysema (Fig. 9.1).

He was treated with a 5-day course of Paxlovid (1 tablet of nirmatrelvir and 1 tablet of ritonavir) starting on the second day of hospitalization, and he was started on amoxicillin and clavulanate potassium to treat his combined bacterial infections. On the third day after admission, his body temperature returned to normal; his oxygen saturation was 100% while on oxygen therapy; his CRP gradually decreased to 76.2 mg/L, and his WBC count decreased to 6.18×10^9/L. Although his infection rapidly resolved, the examination revealed a significant, continuous decrease in hemoglobin. His hemoglobin level was 77 g/L; therefore, the dosage of erythropoietin was increased to 10,000 U twice a week. On the tenth day after admission, his hemoglobin level was 76 g/L, a slight decreased. To prevent a further decrease in hemoglobin, the suspended red blood cells were given. After another 10 days, hemoglobin further decreased to 69 g/L. The possibility of bleeding was ruled out. While he was on anti-infection medication, we switched his anemia medication to roxadustat. Considering the patient's weight, we prescribed a dosage of roxadustat of 100 mg three times a week. The patient's hemoglobin level gradually increased to 94 g/L after 4 weeks (Fig. 9.2).

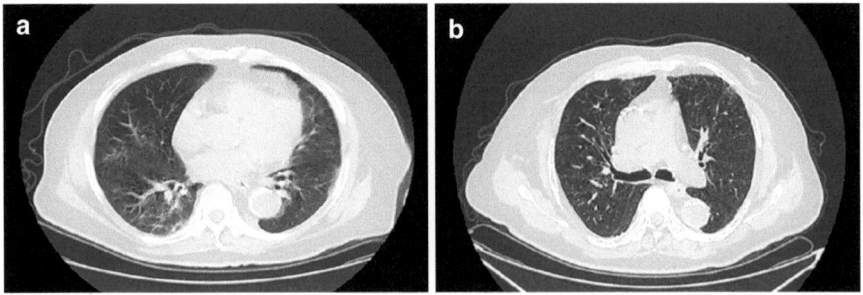

Fig. 9.1 Spiral chest computed tomography (CT) scan indicating multilobular patchy and ground-glass opacities suggestive of COVID-19. (**a**) During COVID-19, (**b**) COVID-19 control

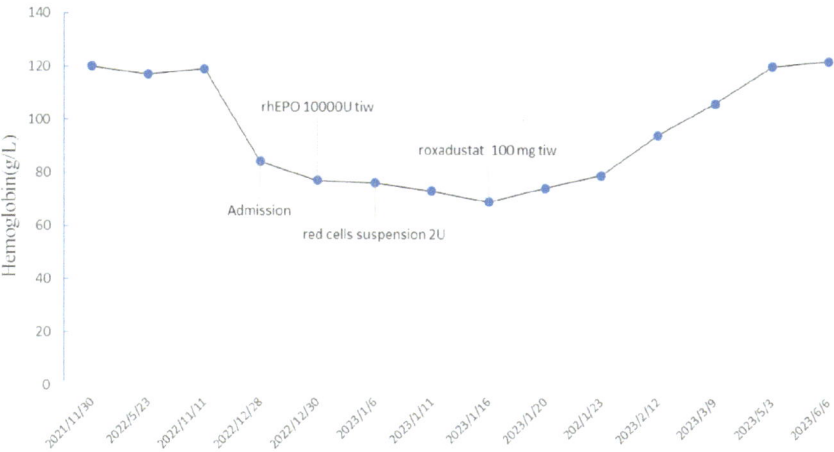

Fig. 9.2 Changes in hemoglobin

9.2   Discussion

The incidence of anemia in dialysis-dependent (DD) patients exceeds 90% [1]. In the past 30 years, the main drugs for treating renal anemia have been erythropoiesis-stimulating agents (ESAs) and iron. The standardized application of an ESA and iron is an important means to improve hemoglobin levels in patients with renal anemia. Therefore, after this patient's admission, we first administered rhEPO and oral iron, which the patient had maintained for a long time and had a good therapeutic effect before he developed COVID-19.

However, this patient's hemoglobin decreased rapidly after COVID-19 pneumonia. It has been reported that the incidence of anemia in hospitalized patients with COVID-19 is approximately 24.7%, and this incidence was associated with advanced age, a decline in renal function, and a high level of inflammation, which are associated with significantly increased levels of inflammatory markers such as CRP or interleukin (IL)-6. Severe anemia significantly increases the mortality of hospitalized patients with COVID-19, although it does not increase the frequency of admission to the intensive care unit (ICU) or the need for mechanical ventilation [2]. Hadadi et al. [3] concluded from their case report that ESA administration to a patient with hypoxic respiratory failure caused by COVID-19 might be the reason for the remission of and final recovery from acute respiratory distress syndrome (ARDS). However, ESA resistance often occurs during infection. Some inflammatory cytokines, such as interleukin-1α (IL-1a), IL-1β, transforming growth factor-β (TGF-β), and tumor necrosis factor-α (TNF-α), can inhibit erythropoietin (EPO) production, downregulate the expression of surface EPO receptors, induce the production of antagonistic peptides that bind to EPO receptors, and inhibit EPO-dependent proliferation [4]. Patients with severe COVID-19 often present with an intense inflammatory phase, which is characterized by a hyperinflammatory state associated with increased concentrations of inflammatory markers such as CRP,

IL-6, and ferritin. This hyperinflammatory state leads to a decrease in circulating iron levels and a decrease in the availability of iron for EPO. In addition, cytokines mediate the inhibition of EPO, shorten the half-life of erythrocytes, and decrease the biological activity of EPO. These factors all limit the efficacy of ESAs, which may at least partly explain why hemoglobin levels continued to decrease in our patient, although we already increased the dose of rh-EPO and injected 2 U of suspended RBCs. There was no evidence of hematological disease or bleeding. This patient's decrease in hemoglobin may have been related to the inflammatory state caused by COVID-19.

Iron is required for an adequate erythropoietic response to rh-EPO. Iron deficiency frequently occurs in patients with chronic kidney disease (CKD) and is mediated by hepcidin, a hepatic peptide that inhibits iron absorption and release from iron stores and macrophages [5]. The production of hepcidin increases during inflammation, which may also lead to ESA resistance because hepcidin directly inhibits the proliferation and survival of erythroid progenitor cells. However, iron is also essential for viral replication and has a potential role in promoting infection. Iron overload can also increase infection risk and worsen CKD-associated inflammation, while inflammation can exacerbate oxidative stress and enhance endothelial dysfunction caused by intravenous (IV) iron administration [6].

This patient had low serum iron and low transferrin saturation; therefore, he was in an iron-deficient state, which might also be the reason for the weak effect of EPO. Clinical judgment is necessary for each individual patient to assess whether there is an immediate need for IV iron, the likelihood of achieving a benefit from a dose of IV iron in the setting of an active infection, and the severity of the infection. Infection may lead to a decrease in circulating iron levels and a decrease in the availability of iron needed for erythropoiesis. Due to this patient's severe COVID-19, we did not administer IV iron therapy.

Hypoxia-inducible factor-prolyl hydroxylase inhibitors (HIF-PHIs) are novel treatments for anemia caused by CKD. HIF-PHIs prevent the degradation of the transcription factor hypoxia-inducible factor. There is evidence to suggest that HIF-PHIs can increase hemoglobin without exacerbating an inflammatory state, making these drugs beneficial for patients in an inflammatory state, especially those with severe infections [7].

In addition to stimulating the production of EPO, HIF-PHIs can improve iron homeostasis and reduce the production of hepcidin in the liver [8], thereby reducing the demand for iron supplementation. In a phase III study of roxadustat in DD-CKD patients in China, similar elevations in hemoglobin levels were observed in patients with normal and elevated CRP levels [9]. For patients in a moderate inflammatory state who may be hyporesponsive to EPO treatment, HIF-PHIs may be an effective alternative to avoid the need for high-dose ESA treatment [10]. There are currently no reports of interactions between roxadustat and Paxlovid, and there was a period of time between the uses of the two drugs in this case. In this patient, hemoglobin steadily increased after his medication regimen was switched to roxadustat, likely because roxadustat can reduce hepcidin, increase iron homeostasis, and increase the sensitivity to EPO.

Here, we report the case of a patient with renal anemia, peritoneal dialysis-dependent CKD, and COVID-19 who was temporarily unsuitable for IV iron therapy and was hyporesponsive to high-dose ESA therapy because of intense inflammation. This case introduces our experience of using an HIF-PHI in such patients. Further research is needed to explore the effectiveness of roxadustat in more COVID-19 patients.

Conflicts We declare that we have no conflicts of interest.

References

1. Evans M, Bower H, Cockburn E, Jacobson SH, Barany P, Carrero JJ. Contemporary management of anaemia, erythropoietin resistance and cardiovascular risk in patients with advanced chronic kidney disease: a nationwide analysis. Clin Kidney J. 2020;13(5):821–7.
2. Bellmann-Weiler R, Lanser L, Barket R, et al. Prevalence and predictive value of anemia and dysregulated iron homeostasis in patients with COVID-19 infection. J Clin Med. 2020;9(8):2429.
3. Hadadi A, Mortezazadeh M, Kolahdouzan K, Alavian G. Does recombinant human erythropoietin administration in critically ill COVID-19 patients have miraculous therapeutic effects? J Med Virol. 2020;92(7):915–8.
4. Portolés J, Martín L, Broseta JJ, Cases A. Anemia in chronic kidney disease: from pathophysiology and current treatments, to future agents. Front Med (Lausanne). 2021;8:642296.
5. Babitt JL, Lin HY. Mechanisms of anemia in CKD. J Am Soc Nephrol. 2012;23(10):1631–4.
6. Macdougall IC, Bircher AJ, Eckardt KU, et al. Iron management in chronic kidney disease: conclusions from a "kidney disease: improving global outcomes" (KDIGO) controversies conference. Kidney Int. 2016;89(1):28–39.
7. Besarab A, Chernyavskaya E, Motylev I, et al. Roxadustat (FG-4592): correction of anemia in incident dialysis patients. J Am Soc Nephrol. 2016;27(4):1225–33.
8. Dhillon S. Roxadustat: first global approval. Drugs. 2019;79(5):563–72.
9. Chen N, Hao C, Liu BC, et al. Roxadustat treatment for anemia in patients undergoing long-term dialysis. N Engl J Med. 2019;381(11):1011–22.
10. Hanna RM, Streja E, Kalantar-Zadeh K. Burden of anemia in chronic kidney disease: beyond erythropoietin. Adv Ther. 2021;38(1):52–75.

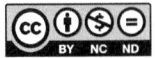

Treatment of Severe Anemia in a Patient with Acute Peritonitis Undergoing Hemodialysis Combined with Peritoneal Dialysis

10

Xiaofei Man, Xiaoyu Xie, and Yan Xu

10.1 Case Presentation

A 36-year-old male was admitted to the hospital on July 11, 2022 due to fever and rash with bilateral lower limb edema. He was diagnosed with systemic lupus erythematosus (SLE) and lupus nephritis 8 years ago. He was treated with prednisone acetate, tacrolimus, and mycophenolate mofetil for 8 years. The patient's serum creatinine started to gradually increase from 6 years ago, reaching 983 μmol/L, and peritoneal dialysis treatment was initiated. Three years prior to admission, the patient suffered from recurrent abdominal pain and was diagnosed with acute peritonitis. In the hospital, he was treated with intra-abdominal gentamicin and vancomycin. Regular hemodialysis treatment supplemented with intermittent peritoneal dialysis was started 2 years ago due to recurrent episodes of peritonitis. Three days prior to admission, the patient experienced another episode of abdominal pain and was treated with antibiotics topically and systemically at the local hospital with no effectiveness.

He had a 5-year history of hypertension with a maximum systolic blood pressure of 220 mmHg and regularly took antihypertensive drugs (valsartan-amlodipine and metoprolol tartrate tablets). The patient also had a 6-year history of bilateral femoral head necrosis and underwent total hip replacement in succession 5 years prior to admission. His vital signs were stable, and his body weight was 70 kg. Physical examination suggested a chronic, anemic appearance, with pale skin and mucous membranes and a tender abdomen with pressure pain and mild rebound pain. No abnormalities were noted on cardiopulmonary examination. One peritoneal dialysis tube was left in the right abdomen.

X. Man · X. Xie · Y. Xu (✉)
Department of Nephrology, The Affiliated Hospital of Qingdao University, Qingdao, China
e-mail: xuyan@qdu.edu.cn

Laboratory examinations (July 12, 2022) revealed a white blood cell (WBC) count of 18.37×10^9/L, a red blood cell (RBC) count of 2.01×10^{12}/L, a hemoglobin concentration of 65 g/L, a platelet (PLT) count of 140×10^9/L, a C-reactive protein (CRP) concentration of 232.8 mg/L, a procalcitonin (PCT) concentration of 4.27 ng/ mL, an albumin concentration of 32 g/L, a blood urea nitrogen concentration of 16.11 mmol/L, a creatinine concentration of 502 μmol/L, a serum potassium concentration of 3.6 mmol/L, a sodium concentration of 138.2 mmol/L, a calcium concentration of 2.24 mmol/L, and a phosphorus concentration of 1.97 mmol/L. Routine examination of ascites fluid showed a muddy appearance, a total cell count of 5978×10^6/L, and a WBC count of 4992×10^6/L. Moreover, anemia-related tests were performed. The tests revealed a ferritin concentration of 407 μg/L, a transferrin saturation of 16.1%, a vitamin B12 concentration of 691 pmol/L, and a folic acid concentration of 27.6 nmol/L. The patient's complement-related tests revealed a complement C3 concentration of 0.8 g/L, a complement C4 concentration of 0.35 g/L, and a parathyroid hormone concentration of 239 ng/L. No other distinguishing abnormalities were observed.

Based on the characteristics of the abovementioned patient, a diagnosis of SLE (lupus nephritis), acute peritonitis, stage 5 chronic kidney disease, renal anemia, secondary hyperparathyroidism, and stage 3 hypertension (very high risk) was made.

After admission, the patient underwent conventional hemodialysis (three times a week for 4 h each session), including hemodialysis filtration and hemoperfusion once every 2 weeks. In addition, he received hemodiafiltration or hemoperfusion once every 2 weeks. To combat infection, the patient was given three types of antibiotics. The treatment plan included 40,000 IU of gentamicin once a day in the abdomen, 500 mg of vancomycin every 5 days in the abdomen, and moxifloxacin (0.4 g once a day via intravenous drop). To treat the primary disease, the medication regimen prescribed for SLE included methylprednisolone 4 mg once a day orally and hydroxychloroquine sulfate 0.2 g once a day orally. In addition to the abovementioned treatments, 0.8 g of sevelamer carbonate was orally administered three times a day to reduce phosphorus levels. Fifteen days after admission, the patient still had severe abdominal pain, and inflammatory indicators such as CRP and PCT had not significantly declined. We then removed the patient's peritoneal dialysis tube on July 26, performing a bacteria culture of the tip of the tube, and the symptoms of abdominal pain were relieved. However, severe abdominal pain occurred 1 day later. Abdominal computed tomography (CT) revealed a large amount of free gas shadow in the abdominal cavity, indicating cavity organ perforation with a large amount of ascites and peritonitis (Figs. 10.1 and 10.2). The patient underwent emergency laparotomy and enterolysis surgery under general anesthesia. Intraoperative exploration revealed a large amount of purulent ascites in the abdominal cavity, similar in appearance to rice water due to the presence of a large amount of pus. After the intestinal adhesions were loosened and thoroughly rinsed, a double tube was placed on both sides of the abdominal wall for later drainage and flushing. Bacterial culture results (July 28, 2022) indicated that the tip of the tube was positive for *Escherichia coli*, and the bacteria were sensitive to meropenem (Fig. 10.3). During the following days, we administered 0.5 g meropenem once every 12 h via

Fig. 10.1 Abdominal CT

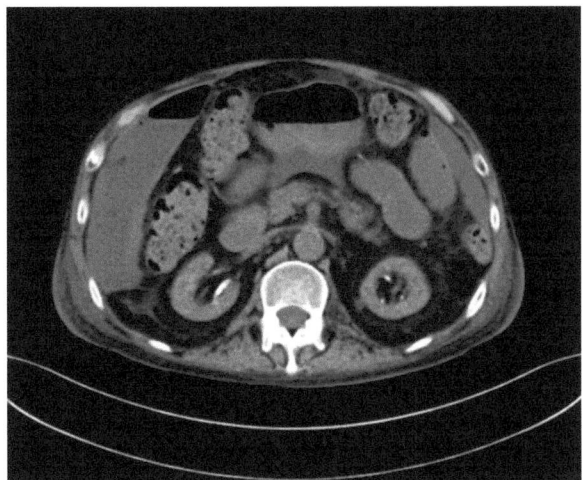

Fig. 10.2 Abdominal CT

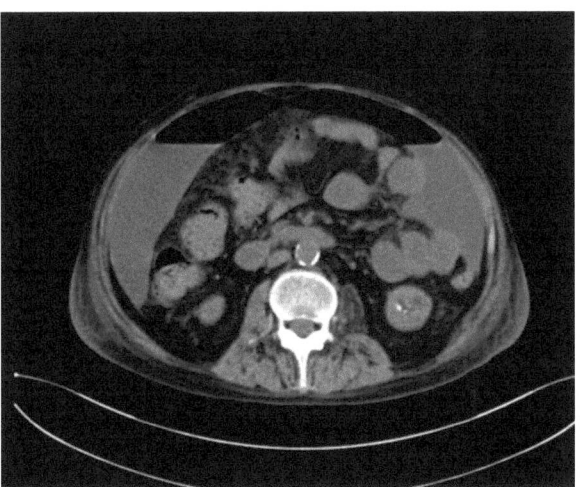

intravenous (IV) injection and repeated peritoneal irrigation. The patient's abdominal pain disappeared, and the inflammatory indicators CRP and PCT gradually decreased with treatment (Figs. 10.4 and 10.5).

Regarding the treatment options and outcomes for patients with renal anemia, our patient's hemoglobin level was 65 g/L upon admission on July 11. Recombinant human erythropoietin (EPO) was intravenously injected at 10,000 IU twice a week, and 9 days after admission, due to severe infection, his hemoglobin decreased to 58 g/L despite the use of a combination of antibiotics and EPO. Between July 21 and July 26, a total of 4 IU of blood was transfused. After hemoglobin reached 70 g/L, the patient underwent peritoneal dialysis tube removal surgery on July 26. The patient then underwent a series of treatments over a period of time, including organ perforation surgery, anti-infection treatment, and repeated abdominal lavage, as

性别 Gender	男 Male	申请病区 Ward	肾病科病区 Department of nephrology	接收时间 Reception time	2022-07-26 16:34
出生日期 Birth	1985-09-22	检验号 Inspection No.	5738923000	报告时间 Report time	2022-07-28 09:01
年龄 Age	36岁	标本 Specimen	导管头 Tip of the tube	报告者 Reporter	彭丽婷
病案号 Medical record No.		医嘱名称 Doctor's advice	细菌培养及鉴定(M 他样本) Bacterial culture and identification	危急说明 Emergency statement	
备注 Note	0				

【历次结果】History of results

项目名称 Test name	代码 Code	结果 Result	单位 Unit	耐药类型 Drug-resistant type	异常提示	参考范围 Reference range	药敏结果	危急提示
项目3	C1402	大肠埃希菌		>15个菌落			药敏结果	
		Escherichia coli		> 15 colonies				

Drug sensitivity results 药敏结果

大肠埃希菌 Escherichia coli

代码 Code	抗生素 Antibiotics	英文名 English name	结果 Results	MIC	mm	用法 Usage	尿液
AMC	阿莫西林-棒醇	Amoxicillin-Clavulanic acid	耐药 Resistance	>=32			
AMK	阿米卡星	Amikacin	敏感 Susceptible	<=2			
AMP	氨苄西林	Ampicillin	耐药 Resistance	>=32			
ATM	氨曲南	Aztreonam	耐药 Resistance	16			
CAZ	头孢他啶	Ceftazidime	耐药 Resistance		12		
CIP	环丙沙星	Ciprofloxacin	耐药 Resistance	>=4			
CRO	头孢曲松	Ceftriaxone	耐药 Resistance	16			
CSL	头孢哌酮/舒巴坦	Cefoperazone/Sulbactam	敏感 Susceptible		23		
CTX	头孢噻肟	Cefotaxime	耐药 Resistance		6		
CXM	头孢呋辛	Cefuroxime	耐药 Resistance		6		
CZO	头孢唑林	Cefazolin	耐药 Resistance	>=64			
ETP	厄他培南	Ertapenem	敏感 Susceptible	<=0.5			
FEP	头孢吡肟	Cefepime	敏感 Susceptible	<=1			
FOX	头孢西丁	Cefoxitin	耐药 Resistance	>=64			
GEN	庆大霉素	Gentamycin	耐药 Resistance	>=16			
IPM	亚胺培南	Imipenem	敏感 Susceptible	<=1			
LVX	左氧氟沙星	Levofloxacin	耐药 Resistance	>=8			
MEM	美罗培南	Meropenem	敏感 Susceptible		28		
SAM	氨苄西林-舒巴坦	Ampicillin-Sulbactam	耐药 Resistance		10		
SXT	复方新诺明	Trimethoprim-Sulfamethoxazole	耐药 Resistance	>=16/304			
TGC	替加环素	Tigecycline	敏感 Susceptible	<=0.5			
TOB	妥布霉素	Tobramycin	中介 Intermediate	8			
TZP	哌拉西林-他唑巴坦	Piperacillin-Tazobactam	敏感 Susceptible	<=4			

Fig. 10.3 Bacterial culture results

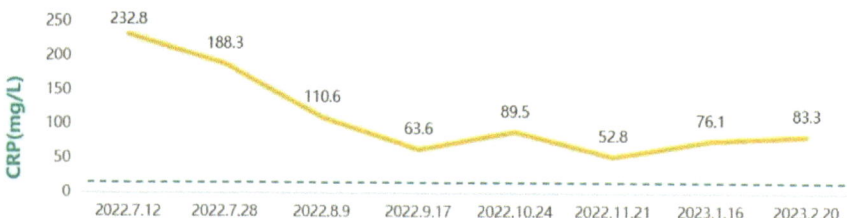

Fig. 10.4 Changes in C-reactive protein levels

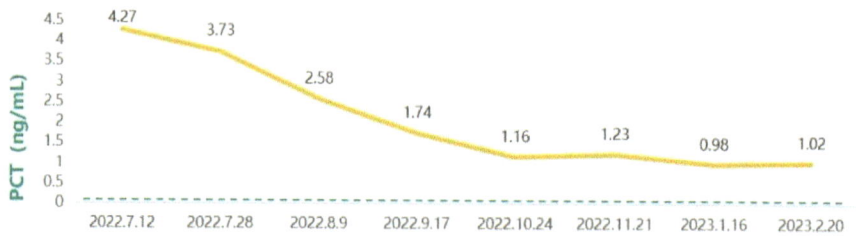

Fig. 10.5 Changes in procalcitonin levels

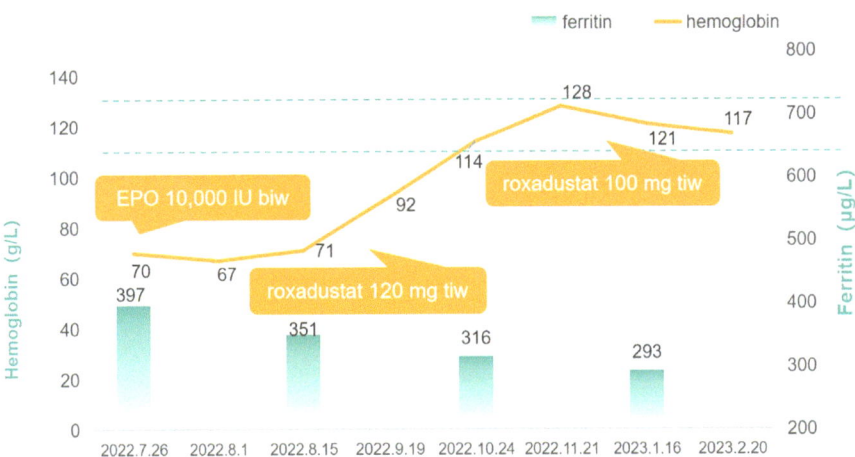

Fig. 10.6 Changes in hemoglobin levels during treatment with different drugs

mentioned earlier, and the inflammation was controlled. Although many efforts were taken as mentioned above, his hemoglobin level only increased slightly even including blood transfusion. His hemoglobin level maintained at 71 g/L; then, we started to use roxadustat on August 15. The initial prescription was roxadustat 120 mg three times a week, and the hemoglobin level increased rapidly within 3 months. After decreasing the roxadustat dosage to 100 mg three times a week, the hemoglobin level showed a downward trend (Fig. 10.6), indicating that roxadustat alleviated renal anemia in a dose-dependent manner. Further dynamic monitoring will be performed to adjust the dosage of roxadustat based on the patient's hemoglobin level.

10.2   Discussion

Anemia is a common complication of chronic kidney disease (CKD) [1], and severe anemia not only increases the risk of cardiovascular issues but also results in significant exhaustion and discomfort, which are historically commonly associated with uremia [2]. Erythropoiesis-stimulating agents (ESAs), in conjunction with iron supplementation, have been the mainstays of treatment for anemia in CKD patients [3]. However, while CKD patients are in an inflammatory state, they are less responsive to ESAs, resulting in renal anemia that is difficult to correct. In inflammatory diseases, cytokines released by activated leukocytes and other cells exert multiple effects that contribute to the reduction in hemoglobin levels through the following pathways:

1. Induction of hepcidin synthesis in the liver (especially by interleukin-6 [IL-6], along with endotoxin). Hepcidin in turn binds to ferroportin, the pore that allows egress of iron from reticuloendothelial macrophages and from intestinal epithelial cells. Binding of hepcidin leads to the internalization and degradation of

ferroportin; the corresponding sequestration of iron within macrophages limits iron availability to erythroid precursors.

2. Inhibition of EPO release from the kidney (especially by interleukin-1β [IL-1β] and tumor necrosis factor α [TNFα]). In turn, EPO-stimulated hematopoietic proliferation is reduced.
3. Direct inhibition of the proliferation of erythroid progenitors (especially by TNFα, interferon-γ [IFNγ], and IL-1β).
4. Augmentation of erythrophagocytosis by reticuloendothelial macrophages (by TNFα) [4]. Iron supplementation may be used to increase iron stores prior to ESA therapy initiation or to improve response to ESA medication to help correct anemia caused by CKD. However, while intravenous injection of iron may be linked to iron overload and associated risks, oral iron is linked to a high rate of gastrointestinal side effects and a high pill burden for patients, leading to adherence concerns.

This patient was diagnosed with lupus nephritis, CKD stage 5, and uremia. He started peritoneal dialysis 6 years prior to admission. Two years prior to admission, he underwent regular hemodialysis as the main mode of dialysis and intermittent peritoneal dialysis as a supplement due to recurrent episodes of peritonitis, and his basic conditions were SLE, hypertension, concomitant renal anemia, hypoproteinemia, hyperphosphatemia, and secondary hyperparathyroidism. He was hospitalized for peritonitis this time. After hospitalization, he actively received treatment, such as anti-infection treatment, blood pressure reducers, systemic lupus erythematosus treatment, and phosphorus reduction. The patient's peritonitis was not well controlled, and he ultimately underwent emergency surgery. Subsequently, anti-infection treatment was continued based on the bacterial culture and drug sensitivity results. After treatment, the patient's inflammatory indicators decreased compared to those before treatment but were still significantly higher than normal. In addition, the patient's renal anemia was not effectively treated with EPO due to the presence of peritonitis. After switching the treatment regimen to roxadustat, the anemia was effectively corrected. Persistent inflammatory state in this patient contributes to the variability in Hb levels and hyporesponsiveness to the ESA. However, hypoxia-inducible factor prolyl hydroxylase inhibitors (HIF-PHIs) can promote endogenous EPO production by activating the HIF pathway and downregulating the HAMP level, wherein efficacy is less affected by inflammation. This may explain the effect of switching to roxadustat.

In this case, the patient's ferritin level was very high, but his transferrin saturation was low, indicating that there was a functional iron deficiency. The patient had inflammation, and excessive iron supplementation aggravated the inflammatory reaction. At the same time, under inflammatory conditions, the EPO response was poor, leading to poor anemia treatment efficacy. After changing the medication to roxadustat, iron utilization increased, which solved the problem of functional iron deficiency, and roxadustat efficacy was not affected by inflammation; therefore, anemia was significantly ameliorated.

HIF-PHIs represent a promising new class of orally administered drugs currently used for the treatment of anemia in CKD patients [1, 5]. A study showed that for nondialysis-dependent chronic kidney disease (NDD-CKD) patients, HIF-PHIs could relieve functional iron deficiency by promoting iron transport and utilization, which may be achieved by lowering hepcidin levels [6]. In addition, HIF-PHIs have heterogeneous effects on iron metabolism. HIF-PHIs activate the HIF oxygen-sensing pathway and are effective in correcting and maintaining hemoglobin levels in patients with nondialysis- and dialysis-dependent CKD [7]. Some data also suggest that the efficacy of HIF-PHIs and, consequently, the dose needs, are less influenced by inflammation than are those of ESAs [8]. Roxadustat is an HIF-PHI that increases hemoglobin by stimulating EPO synthesis and increasing iron availability through the facilitation of iron uptake and/or release from stores. When combined with the oral administration of roxadustat, which is normally delivered in centers, a reduced need for intravenous iron therapy may support the management of CKD-related anemia at home [9]. In this case, roxadustat can correct refractory anemia caused by ESA resistance, and roxadustat efficacy is not affected by inflammatory status. In this case, the effect of roxadustat was dose dependent. When the patient was given a dosage of 120 mg three times a week, hemoglobin levels increased rapidly within 3 months, but after decreasing the dosage to 100 mg three times a week, hemoglobin levels showed a downward trend. These results suggested that the dosage of HIF-PHI should be adjusted according to the fluctuations in hemoglobin.

References

1. Ikeda Y. Novel roles of HIF-PHIs in chronic kidney disease: the link between iron metabolism, kidney function, and FGF23. Kidney Int. 2021;100(1):14–6.
2. Locatelli F, Del Vecchio L. Quality of life: a crucial aspect for the patients, a neglected goal in the treatment of anemia in patients with CKD. Kidney Int. 2023;103(6):1025–7.
3. Sugahara M, Tanaka T, Nangaku M. Future perspectives of anemia management in chronic kidney disease using hypoxia-inducible factor-prolyl hydroxylase inhibitors. Pharmacol Ther. 2022;239:108272.
4. Zarychanski R, Houston DS. Anemia of chronic disease: a harmful disorder or an adaptive, beneficial response? CMAJ. 2008;179(4):333–7.
5. Ku E, Del Vecchio L, Eckardt KU, et al. Novel anemia therapies in chronic kidney disease: conclusions from a kidney disease: improving global outcomes (KDIGO) controversies conference. Kidney Int. 2023;104(4):655–80.
6. Yang J, Xing J, Zhu X, Xie X, Wang L, Zhang X. Effects of hypoxia-inducible factor-prolyl hydroxylase inhibitors vs. erythropoiesis-stimulating agents on iron metabolism in non-dialysis-dependent anemic patients with CKD: a network meta-analysis. Front Endocrinol (Lausanne). 2023;14:1131516.
7. Pergola PE, Charytan C, Little DJ, et al. Changes in iron availability with roxadustat in nondialysis-and dialysis-dependent patients with anemia of CKD. Kidney360. 2022;3(9):1511–28.
8. Locatelli F, Del Vecchio L. Hypoxia-inducible factor-prolyl hydroxyl domain inhibitors: from theoretical superiority to clinical noninferiority compared with current ESAs? J Am Soc Nephrol. 2022;33(11):1966–79.
9. Souza E, Cho KH, Harris ST, Flindt NR, Watt RK, Pai AB. Hypoxia-inducible factor prolyl hydroxylase inhibitors: a paradigm shift for treatment of anemia in chronic kidney disease? Expert Opin Investig Drugs. 2020;29(8):831–44.

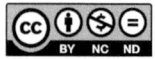

COVID-19 Exacerbated Renal Anemia in a Maintenance Hemodialysis Patient

11

Xiao Liu and San-Tao Ou

11.1 Case Presentation

A 72-year-old man had been suffering from uremia for 11 years and was receiving hemodialysis three times a week. He was diagnosed with renal anemia, for which he was treated by subcutaneous injections of erythropoiesis-stimulating agents (ESAs) and roxadustat. Five months earlier, due to unsatisfactory correction of anemia, he received ESAs at doses of 9000 U once a week, together with roxadustat at a dose of 100 mg three times a week for treating anemia. His hemoglobin concentrations gradually rose to 12.2 g/dl.

He unfortunately suffered from COVID-19 and tested positive for nucleic acid. During this period, hemoglobin showed a decreasing trend, reaching a minimum of 5.5 g/dL. Then, under regular dialysis, the dose of ESAs was adjusted to 6000 U three times a week combined with 150 mg roxadustat three times a week. Despite the aforementioned treatment, his anemia remained uncorrected, necessitating repeated blood transfusions to improve his anemic condition (total blood transfused: 1900 ml), with hemoglobin levels fluctuating between 5.0 and 7.9 g/dL. To explore the cause of anemia, comprehensive assessments were conducted, including hematological indices, autoantibodies, viral infections (hepatitis B and C, as well as HIV), serum protein electrophoresis, immunofixation electrophoresis, and Coombs tests. No significant abnormal findings were observed. An abdominal CT scan did not reveal splenomegaly. Thus, to determine the etiology of his anemia, a bone marrow puncture was performed, revealing features consistent with proliferative anemia and no other conspicuous abnormalities. Following the exclusion of other causes of anemia, we hypothesized a potential association between anemia and COVID-19.

X. Liu · S.-T. Ou (✉)
Department of Nephrology, The Affiliated Hospital of Southwest Medical University, Luzhou, Sichuan Province, China

© The Author(s) 2025
B.-C. Liu (ed.), *Treatment of Refractory Renal Anemia*,
https://doi.org/10.1007/978-981-97-7636-8_11

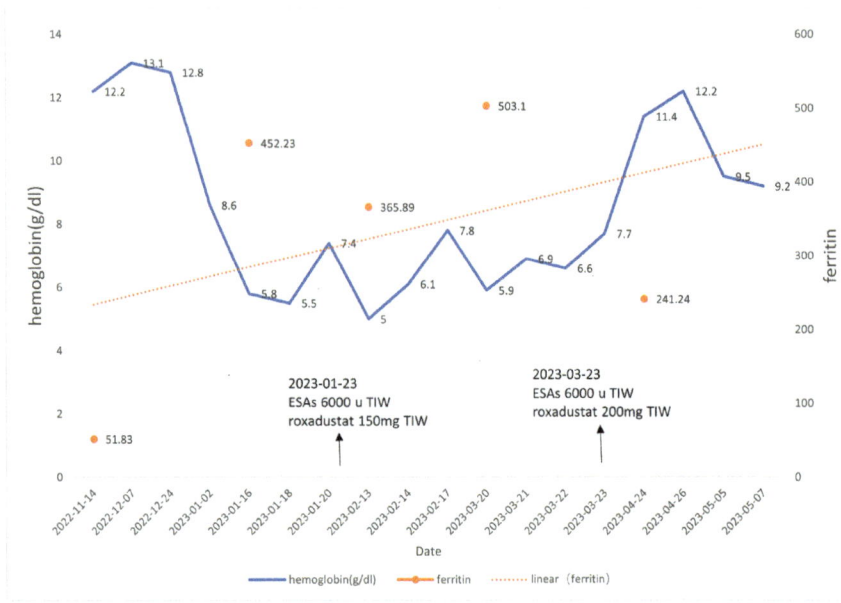

Fig. 11.1 Changes in hemoglobin and ferritin levels

He had a 20-year history of diabetes, necessitating subcutaneous administration of recombinant insulin. Additionally, he has a 10-year history of hypertension and has been on long-term medication with nifedipine controlled-release tablet, which is an antihypertensive agent.

After repeated transfusions and taking into account the patient's medical history, we adjusted the dosage of ESAs to 6000 U three times a week, in conjunction with roxadustat at a dose of 200 mg three times a week. During the 2-month follow-up, the patient's hemoglobin level stayed within the range of 8.0–12.2 g/dL (Fig. 11.1).

11.2   Discussion

In this study, we report on an elderly male patient who underwent regular hemodialysis and had a history of type 2 diabetes and hypertension. Before hospitalization, he had been receiving high-dose ESAs in combination with roxadustat, which kept his hemoglobin stable. However, the patient was infected with COVID-19, prompting adjustments to the anemia management regimen. The dosage of ESAs was increased to 6000 U three times a week, along with roxadustat at a dosage of 150 mg three times weekly. Even with the abovementioned treatment, anemia persisted and required blood transfusion. After repeated blood transfusions, although his hemoglobin remained low, the patient's anemia symptoms significantly improved. Therefore, the notable feature of this case was the exacerbation of stable anemia due to COVID-19 under combined treatment with ESAs and roxadustat.

Anemia is a common complication in patients with chronic kidney disease (CKD), profoundly impacting their quality of life and facilitating the progression of CKD. Its pathogenesis primarily involves diminished endogenous ESA production, along with factors such as inflammation, a shortened red blood cell lifespan, and uremic toxins. Traditional therapeutic approaches include the use of iron supplements, ESAs, and, when necessary, blood transfusions. In recent years, HIF-α prolyl hydroxylase inhibitors (HIF-PHIs) have emerged as novel drugs for the management of renal anemia [1–4].

In clinical practice, ESAs have long been the mainstay for treating renal anemia. Their therapeutic efficacy is influenced by numerous factors, such as inflammation, iron deficiency, secondary hyperparathyroidism (SHPT), inadequate dialysis, and chronic bleeding [4]. Roxadustat, a prolyl hydroxylase inhibitor, can simulate a hypoxic environment, thereby promoting the endogenous production of erythropoietin (EPO) and its receptor (EPOR), leading to the amelioration of anemia [2]. A study focusing on dialysis patients reported that roxadustat is as effective as ESA [5]. Furthermore, in other relevant studies, its efficacy remains unaffected by the level of inflammation, and it can improve iron homeostasis [2, 6]. Hence, roxadustat serves as an alternative treatment for patients who respond poorly to ESAs.

The patient in this case had been receiving ESA therapy for 2 years with unsatisfactory increases in hemoglobin. After excluding potential factors contributing to his poor response to ESA, we started him on a combination of ESA (with dosage adjustments based on hemoglobin levels) and roxadustat (100 mg three times weekly), and this gradually stabilized his hemoglobin levels. However, the patient was infected with COVID-19 approximately 5 months earlier, prompting a comprehensive set of relevant ancillary investigations. We combined the inspection results and then considered the exacerbation of anemia attributable to COVID-19.

Recent studies have indicated a close association between COVID-19 and anemia [7, 8]. In the pathogenesis of COVID-19, systemic inflammation plays a crucial role in disease progression. Elevated expression [8–10] of proinflammatory cytokines such as IFN-γ, TNF-α, and IL-6 (with SARS-CoV-2 stimulating IL-6 production by binding to macrophage ACE2 receptors) is observed, with IL-6 playing a central role in the cytokine storm [10–12]. Additionally, IL-6, a pleiotropic cytokine, increases hepcidin levels and induces iron-restricted erythropoiesis and inflammatory anemia via the IL-6/STAT3 pathway [8, 13, 14]. Here, we define inflammatory anemia as normocytic normochromic anemia with evidence of inflammation and iron restriction not attributed to systemic iron deficiency [15]. The pathogenesis of inflammatory anemia may involve the following aspects([10, 14–16]: (1) Iron, as one of the essential raw materials for hematopoiesis, exhibits inhibitory effects on red blood cell production due to macrophage iron sequestration and reduced intestinal iron absorption during inflammation. Studies suggest that anemia in COVID-19 patients may result from altered iron metabolism and iron-restricted erythropoiesis [17]. (2) In an inflammatory environment, the generation or activity of erythropoietin may be suppressed, leading to a diminished response to anemia. (3) Inflammatory cytokines can shorten the lifespan of red blood cells and inhibit their differentiation. Research indicated [8] that increased expression of proinflammatory cytokines such as IFN-γ or TNF-α in COVID-19 patients can impact erythropoiesis or the half-life of red blood cells. Evidence [9] has shown that 56.0% to 68.8% of anemic patients admitted with COVID-19 exhibited features of inflammatory anemia, and among subjects hospitalized for at least 2 weeks, the prevalence of anemia reaches 87.8%, which is often characterized by elevated levels of the iron storage protein ferritin and decreased circulating iron availability. In the current patient, following the infection with COVID-19, there was a concurrence between the increase in ferritin levels and the decline in hemoglobin. This phenomenon was also observed in a meta-analysis [17], in which COVID-19 patients often exhibited hypochromic anemia and hyperferritinemia. Additionally, the presence of newly developed anemia strongly reflects the progression of inflammation-related diseases [9], and the severity of anemia is positively correlated with the level of inflammation [11]. Particularly, inflammatory anemia is widely observed in individuals severely infected with SARS-CoV-2 [16].

This case report describes a worsening of stable anemia due to COVID-19 under combined treatment with EPO and roxadustat. Following the patient's COVID-19 infection, there was a significant decrease in hemoglobin levels. Despite repeated blood transfusions, the hemoglobin level remained low, fluctuating around 5.0–7.9 g/dL. There is growing evidence of potentially harmful effects of blood transfusions, such as secondary iron overload, liver cirrhosis, cardiomyopathy, eventual damage to multiple organs, and even death. The guiding principle for transfusion therapy should be "less is more" [15]. Therefore, we adjusted the treatment regimen to include an ESA dose of 6000 U TIW in combination with roxadustat at a dose of 200 mg three times a week. Two months after, the patient's hemoglobin levels have remained stable between 8.0 and 12.2 g/dL, resulting in a significant improvement in the symptoms of anemia and reduced reliance on blood transfusions.

References

1. Cases A, Egocheaga MI, Tranche S, et al. Anemia of chronic kidney disease: protocol of study, management and referral to Nephrology. Aten Primaria. 2018;50(1):60–4.
2. Liu J, Yang F, Waheed Y, Li S, Liu K, Zhou X. The role of roxadustat in chronic kidney disease patients complicated with anemia. Korean J Intern Med. 2023;38(2):147–56.
3. Weir MR. Managing anemia across the stages of kidney disease in those hyporesponsive to erythropoiesis-stimulating agents. Am J Nephrol. 2021;52(6):450–66.
4. Zhong H, Lin W, Zhou T. Current and emerging drugs in the treatment of anemia in patients with chronic kidney disease. J Pharm Pharm Sci. 2020;23:278–88.
5. Chen N, Hao C, Liu BC, et al. Roxadustat treatment for anemia in patients undergoing long-term dialysis. N Engl J Med. 2019;381(11):1011–22.
6. Raichoudhury R, Spinowitz BS. Treatment of anemia in difficult-to-manage patients with chronic kidney disease. Kidney Int Suppl (2011). 2021;11(1):26–34.
7. Chen C, Zhou W, Fan W, et al. Association of anemia and COVID-19 in hospitalized patients. Future Virol. 2021; https://doi.org/10.2217/fvl-2021-0044.
8. Bergamaschi G, De Andreis FB, Aronico N, et al. Anemia in patients with COVID-19: pathogenesis and clinical significance. Clin Exp Med. 2021;21(2):239–46.

9. Lanser L, Burkert FR, Bellmann-Weiler R, et al. Dynamics in anemia development and dysregulation of iron homeostasis in hospitalized patients with COVID-19. Meta. 2021;11(10):653.

10. Fouad SH, Allam MF, Taha SI, et al. Comparison of hemoglobin level and neutrophil to lymphocyte ratio as prognostic markers in patients with COVID-19. J Int Med Res. 2021;49(7):3000605211030124.

11. Tao Z, Xu J, Chen W, et al. Anemia is associated with severe illness in COVID-19: a retrospective cohort study. J Med Virol. 2021;93(3):1478–88.

12. Zhang C, Wu Z, Li JW, Zhao H, Wang GQ. Cytokine release syndrome in severe COVID-19: interleukin-6 receptor antagonist tocilizumab may be the key to reduce mortality. Int J Antimicrob Agents. 2020;55(5):105954.

13. Camaschella C, Nai A, Silvestri L. Iron metabolism and iron disorders revisited in the hepcidin era. Haematologica. 2020;105(2):260–72.

14. Weiss G, Ganz T, Goodnough LT. Anemia of inflammation. Blood. 2019;133(1):40–50.

15. Ganz T. Anemia of inflammation. N Engl J Med. 2019;381(12):1148–57.

16. Bellmann-Weiler R, Lanser L, Barket R, et al. Prevalence and predictive value of anemia and dysregulated iron homeostasis in patients with COVID-19 infection. J Clin Med. 2020;9(8):2429.

17. Taneri PE, Gómez-Ochoa SA, Llanaj E, et al. Anemia and iron metabolism in COVID-19: a systematic review and meta-analysis. Eur J Epidemiol. 2020;35(8):763–73.

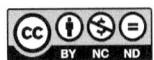

Treatment of Anemia Complicated with Severe Infection in a Hemodialysis Patient

Liangying Gan and Li Zuo

12.1 Case Presentation

A 43-year-old male who complained of "hematuria and proteinuria for 9 years, maintenance hemodialysis for 7 years, and fever for 4 days" was admitted in July 2019.

The patient presented with hematuria and proteinuria 9 years ago and was diagnosed with chronic glomerulonephritis, IgA nephropathy, and renal hypertension by renal biopsy. Seven years ago, maintenance hemodialysis was started; high-flux dialysis was performed twice a week; hemodiafiltration was performed once a week; and the urea clearance index (Kt/v) was kept above 1.2 for the past 3 months. The patient took lanthanum carbonate for a long time to reduce his serum phosphorus and calcitriol to correct secondary hyperparathyroidism and was given amlodipine and Betaloc to lower his blood pressure. The patient did not use erythropoiesis-stimulating drugs in the past 3 months. His dry weight was 77 kg; blood pressure was mostly maintained at 110 ~ 130/(75 ~ 85) mmHg; hemoglobin stayed within 110 ~ 115 g/L; albumin was 40 ~ 42 g/L; serum calcium was 2.4 ~ 2.5 mmol/L; serum phosphorus was 1.42 ~ 1.67 mmol/L; and parathyroid hormone was 126.1 ~ 257.6 pg/ml. Four days before admission, the patient developed fever and chills after catching a cold on exertion, especially at night, sometimes with headache, mild suffocation, fatigue, and anorexia, and he intermittently took ibuprofen orally.

Antipyretic treatment: Two days before admission, the patient developed chills during dialysis, with a body temperature of 39.2 °C and a decrease in blood pressure to 85/54 mmHg, which improved after termination of dialysis and symptomatic and supportive treatment. The patient was given anti-infective treatment with ertapenem

L. Gan (✉) · L. Zuo
Department of Nephrology, Peking University People's Hospital, Beijing, China
e-mail: ganl@bjmu.edu.cn

© The Author(s) 2025
B.-C. Liu (ed.), *Treatment of Refractory Renal Anemia*,
https://doi.org/10.1007/978-981-97-7636-8_12

and moxifloxacin in the emergency department for 2 days, and his symptoms did not significantly improve. The patient was then admitted to the hospital.

He denied any history of diabetes or coronary heart disease. He had an arteriovenous fistula in his left forearm. He denied any history of food or drug allergy. His parents suffered from hypertension and denied a family history of genetic diseases.

Physical examination showed his temperature was 39.5 °C; pulse was 130 beats/minute; respiratory rate was 30 breaths/minute; and blood pressure was 150/77 mmHg. His consciousness was clear; the breath sounds in both lungs were coarse; and moist rales could be heard in the right lower lung. The rest of the physical examination was unremarkable.

Laboratory examination showed the following: the white blood cell count was 14.2×10^9/L, neutrophil percentage 83.2%, hemoglobin 113 g/L, C-reactive protein 239.89 mg/L, and procalcitonin 27.07 µg/L. Blood gas analysis revealed the following: pH 7.44, oxygen partial pressure 62 mmHg, carbon dioxide pressure 40 mmHg, oxygen saturation 92%, serum sodium 126 mmol/L, and lactate 2.8 mmol/L. Blood culture was negative. Chest CT showed multiple infections in both lungs, bilateral pleural effusion with partial atelectasis of adjacent lung tissues, and interstitial effusion in both lungs. Bronchoscopy showed endobronchial inflammatory changes, but etiological examination of bronchoalveolar lavage fluid by bronchoscopy was negative. Echocardiography showed no valvular vegetations.

The main clinical diagnoses are the following:

1. Chronic renal failure (maintenance hemodialysis).
    Chronic glomerulonephritis (IgA nephropathy)
    Renal anemia
    Renal hypertension
    Mineral and bone disorders in chronic kidney disease
2. Double-lung pneumonia
    Bilateral pleural effusion
    Respiratory failure (type I)

Clinical treatment process: After admission, he was given active anti-infective treatment and empirical medication covering common pathogens. The specific medication regimen was as follows: Cefoperazone/sulbactam 3 g once a day combined with moxifloxacin 400 mg once a day for 3 days; meropenem 0.5 g once a day combined with azithromycin 0.5 g once a day for 7 days; meropenem 0.5 g once a day combined with linezolid 600 mg twice a day for 4 days; and linezolid 600 mg once a day for 3 days supplemented with symptomatic and supportive treatment. After 17 days of adequate anti-infective treatment, the patient's body temperature

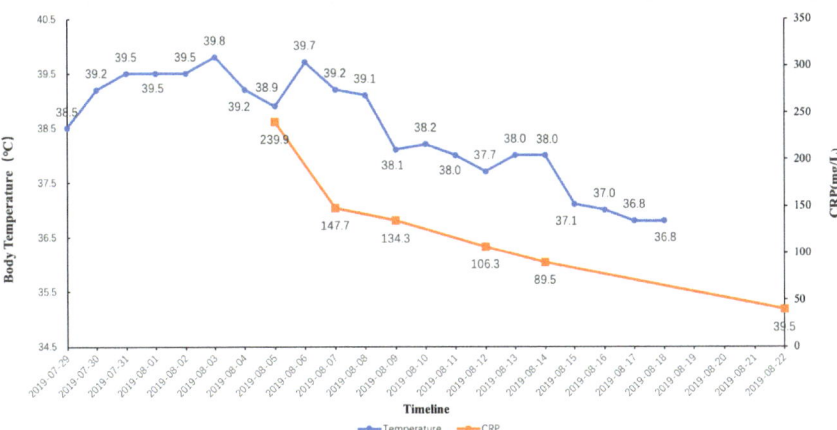

Fig. 12.1 Changes in body temperature and C-reactive protein levels during anti-infection treatment

returned to normal, and the inflammatory indicators showed decreasing trends. The changes in body temperature and C-reactive protein during treatment are shown in Fig. 12.1. During this period, hemoglobin was reviewed several times, and it progressively decreased. On August 7, 2019, hemoglobin (92 g/L) was re-examined, and 3000 U of erythropoiesis-stimulating agent (ESA) was added three times a week via subcutaneous injection. His hemoglobin was re-examined several times and still showed a decreasing trend. On August 22, 2019, hemoglobin decreased to 73 g/L. To further correct his anemia, he took 120 mg roxadustat orally three times a week. Thereafter, the patient's lowest hemoglobin concentration decreased to 65 g/L. On September 21, 2019, after 4 weeks of roxadustat use, hemoglobin increased to 81 g/L, so the dose of roxadustat was reduced to 100 mg three times a week.

On October 22, hemoglobin was 99 g/L, and the patient's anemia was basically corrected. The therapeutic drug was replaced with ESA (3000 U) three times a week subcutaneously, and the patient's hemoglobin level remained stable. Changes in hemoglobin during treatment are shown in Fig. 12.2.

Ferritin increased from 224.9 µg/L before infection (June 17, 2019) to 538.7 µg/L during infection (August 22, 2019), and iron supplementation was not given. After the infection was corrected, it decreased to 58 µg/L during roxadustat treatment (October 10, 2019), and a continuous intravenous drip of 100 mg of iron sucrose every 2 weeks was started.

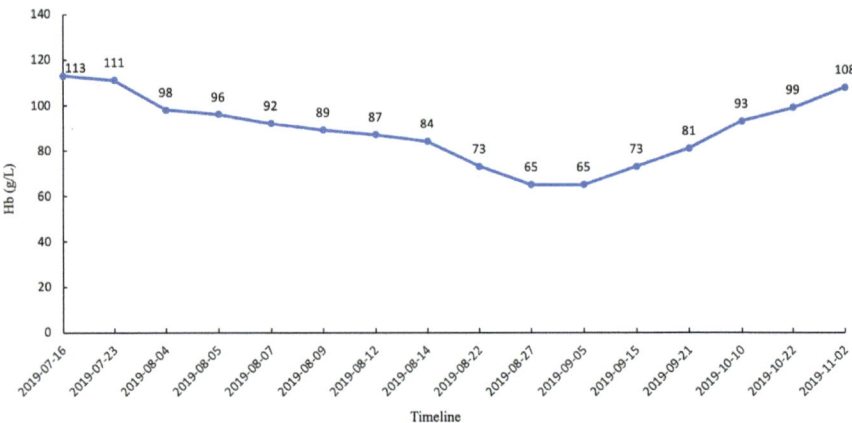

Fig. 12.2 Changes in hemoglobin and use of anti-anemia drugs. Note: From July 16 to August 6, 2019, the patient did not receive anti-anemia treatment; from August 7 to 21, 2019, the patient was treated with ESA at a dose of 3000 U subcutaneously three times a week; from August 22 to September 20, 2019, the patient was switched to roxadustat 120 mg, orally, three times a week; from September 21 to October 21, 2019, the dose of roxadustat was reduced to 100 mg three times a week; from October 22 to November 2, 2019, the patient was switched back to ESA 3000 U subcutaneously three times a week

12.2   Discussion

This patient was a middle-aged male with a chronic course and acute exacerbation. The patient's previous dialysis condition was stable, and various complications clinically improved after treatment. His lungs became infected after exertion; the infection progressed rapidly, and respiratory failure and hypotension occurred 2 days later. After 3 weeks of active anti-infective treatment, the patient's clinical symptoms were relieved, and his body temperature returned to normal. Hemoglobin progressively decreased from 113 g/L to 65 g/L within 1 month, and under the premise of active control of infection, hemoglobin still progressively decreased after routine application of EPO to correct anemia. Four weeks after switching to roxadustat, hemoglobin increased by 16 g/L, and 8 weeks after use, hemoglobin increased by 34 g/L, and his anemia was gradually corrected. During the severe infection, ferritin significantly increased, but after infection was controlled and during the improvement in hemoglobin synthesis with roxadustat, ferritin significantly decreased (from 538.7 µg/L to 58 µg/L), reaching the level of iron deficiency in dialysis patients and required timely iron supplementation.

Inflammation is common in patients with end-stage renal disease (ESRD), being present in 30% to 60% of dialysis patients in North America and Europe, and is associated with many factors, such as uremic toxin accumulation, oxygenation stress response, and protein-energy wasting (PEW) and infection. Dialysis patients are prone to infection due to immune dysfunction and a variety of complications, and infection can lead to the occurrence and progression of a variety of complications and is also one of the leading causes of death in dialysis patients [1].

Anemia in patients with chronic kidney disease (CKD) is multifactorial. Inflammatory states such as infection can lead to the activation of monocytes and T cells and the release of cytokines such as interferon-γ (IFN-γ), tumor necrosis factor-α (TNF-α), interleukin-1β (IL-1β), and IL-6, which, in turn, lead to the occurrence or aggravation of anemia through a variety of mechanisms, including the following: (1) TNF-α, IFN-γ, and IL-1β directly inhibit the proliferation of erythroid progenitor cells. (2) IL-1β and TNF-α inhibit the release of EPO from the kidney, which then inhibits the process of EPO-stimulated hematopoietic proliferation. (3) IL-6 and endotoxin can induce the synthesis of hepatic hepcidin, which, in turn, affects the transport of intracellular iron to the circulation. (4) Lastly, TNF-α can enhance erythrocyte phagocytosis of the reticuloendothelial system, such as macrophages [2, 3]. Thus, infection increases erythrocyte destruction and thus affects the whole process of bone marrow hematopoiesis, from the differentiation and proliferation of bone marrow erythroid progenitor cells to the EPO-dependent stage to the iron-dependent stage.

In this maintenance hemodialysis patient, hemoglobin progressively decreased, and anemia became aggravated after severe infection. The addition of 3000 U ESA three times a week did not improve anemia, which could be related to the fact that the patient's infection was not well controlled. In hemodialysis patients, it is noted that the higher the CRP level, the lower the hemoglobin despite a higher dose of ESA. This finding suggests that in the inflammatory state, ESA had an unsatisfactory effect on the blood [4].

Hypoxia-inducible factor (HIF) is a transcription factor that responds to decreased oxygen concentrations by activating the expression of specific genes to maintain physiological homeostasis. HIF is a heterodimer consisting of an oxygen-sensing alpha-subunit and a constitutively expressed beta-subunit [5]. At normal oxygen concentrations, the proline group on HIF-α is hydroxylated by HIF prolyl hydroxylase (HIF-PH) and degraded. HIF-PHI mimics the inhibition of HIF-PH in a hypoxic environment and prevents HIF-PH from degrading HIF-α, thereby initiating the HIF pathway and regulating downstream genes. On the one hand, the regulation of erythropoiesis increases EPO and EPO receptor production. On the other hand, the regulation of iron metabolism, including decreasing hepcidin levels and increasing the expression of divalent metal ion transporter (DMT1), duodenal cytochrome B (DcytB), transferrin, and transferrin receptor, improves anemia [6].

In a phase III clinical study of dialysis patients in China, after stratification according to whether the baseline C-reactive protein level was higher than the upper limit of normal, the dose of HIF-PHI roxadustat and the hemoglobin level were comparable between the groups with normal and elevated CRP. In the EPO group, as in the aforementioned studies, hemoglobin levels were still lower than those in the normal CRP group even at higher doses in dialysis patients with CRP above the upper limit of normal [7], suggesting that roxadustat has a better corrective effect on anemia in patients with inflammation than without inflammation. The effect of HIF-PHI on iron metabolism may be one of the mechanisms by which it improves the condition of patients with infection or inflammation. HIF pathway activation can not only increase intestinal iron absorption but also reduce hepcidin levels and facilitate iron utilization in the body.

Hepcidin is an endogenous antimicrobial polypeptide synthesized and secreted by hepatocytes. When the body's iron level increases or inflammation and infection occur, the body's hepcidin level is upregulated, but its expression is downregulated when hypoxia, anemia, or EPO increases [8]. Hepcidin binds to membrane iron transporters in vivo, internalizes into cells, and is degraded by lysosomes. Membrane iron transporters, on the other hand, are the main iron export proteins that transport iron absorbed by intestinal epithelial cells into the circulation and allow macrophages to recycle and transport iron from damaged erythrocytes into the circulation. During inflammation or infection, hepcidin increases, and its inhibitory effect on membrane iron transporters prevents the transfer of intracellular iron to the extracellular space. Nemeth et al. showed that after exogenous infusion of IL-6 in normal humans, hepcidin levels were significantly higher in vivo, while serum iron and transferrin saturation decreased [9]. Compared with ESA, roxadustat significantly reduced hepcidin levels. This effect may be one of the mechanisms by which roxadustat can exert a better blood-raising effect during inflammation [7, 10].

In this case, although ESA was not used within 3 months before infection, hemoglobin was still maintained at 113 g/L, suggesting that the patient had a certain amount of EPO synthesis. As mentioned earlier, it is speculated that, on the one hand, EPO synthesis may decrease during infection, and even if it does not decrease, the level of EPO is no longer high enough to maintain the patient's hemoglobin level. Meanwhile, on the other hand, during inflammation, a larger dose of ESA still cannot improve the blood-raising effect, so after the addition of ESA therapy in this patient, hemoglobin continued to decrease. Switching to roxadustat can significantly increase hemoglobin, which is related to the good control of the infection and may also be related to the fact that roxadustat has multiple blood-increasing mechanisms, especially the downregulation of hepcidin during inflammation and the improvement of iron metabolism.

References

1. Zimmermann J, Herrlinger S, Pruy A, Metzger T, Wanner C. Inflammation enhances cardiovascular risk and mortality in hemodialysis patients. Kidney Int. 1999;55(2):648–58.
2. Zarychanski R, Houston DS. Anemia of chronic disease: a harmful disorder or an adaptive, beneficial response? CMAJ. 2008;179(4):333–7.
3. Hom J, Dulmovits BM, Mohandas N, Blanc L. The erythroblastic Island as an emerging paradigm in the anemia of inflammation. Immunol Res. 2015;63:75–89.
4. Bradbury BD, Critchlow CW, Weir MR, Stewart R, Krishnan M, Hakim RH. Impact of elevated C-reactive protein levels on erythropoiesis- stimulating agent (ESA) dose and responsiveness in hemodialysis patients. Nephrol Dial Transplant. 2009;24(3):919–25.
5. Semenza GL. Targeting HIF-1 for cancer therapy. Nat Rev Cancer. 2003;3(10):721–32.
6. Locatelli F, Fishbane S, Block GA, Macdougall IC. Targeting hypoxia-inducible factors for the treatment of anemia in chronic kidney disease patients. Am J Nephrol. 2017;45(3):187–99.

7. Chen N, Hao C, Liu BC, et al. Roxadustat treatment for anemia in patients undergoing long-term dialysis. N Engl J Med. 2019;381(11):1011–22.
8. Nemeth E, Rivera S, Gabayan V, et al. IL-6 mediates hypoferremia of inflammation by inducing the synthesis of the iron regulatory hormone hepcidin. J Clin Investig. 2004;113(9):1271–6.
9. Piperno A, Galimberti S, Mariani R, et al. Modulation of hepcidin production during hypoxia-induced erythropoiesis in humans in vivo: data from the HIGHCARE project. Blood J Am Soc Hematol. 2011;117(10):2953–9.
10. Chen N, Qian J, Chen J, et al. Phase 2 studies of oral hypoxia-inducible factor prolyl hydroxylase inhibitor FG-4592 for treatment of anemia in China. Nephrol Dial Transplant. 2017;32(8):1373–86.

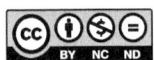

Treatment of Renal Anemia in a Maintenance Hemodialysis Patient with Viral Hepatitis B Infection

13

Li Chen and Wen-Xiu Chang

13.1 Case Presentation

The patient was a 40-year-old male who had elevated serum creatinine for 9 years before admission. He had a history of hypertension for more than 20 years and gout for 10 years. Meanwhile, he was positive for chronic hepatitis B virus infection (HBsAg, HBeAg, and anti-HBc positive) and was obese as well (height: 175 cm, body weight: 110 kg). Initially, his serum creatinine was approximately 380 μmol/L, but he did not give it enough attention. Five years before admission, he had a bout of vomiting composed of gastric contents accompanied by edema throughout the body. Upon examination at a local hospital, the patient's serum creatinine was 1188 μmol/L, and his symptoms did not improve after symptomatic treatment. He was referred to the department of nephrology of our hospital. He had a hemoglobin level of 76 g/L, a serum creatinine level of 1194 μmol/L, a carbon dioxide-binding capacity of 15.9 mmol/L, a blood potassium concentration of 5.41 mmol/L, a blood calcium concentration of 1.25 mmol/L, and a blood phosphorus concentration of 2.59 mmol/L. Urinary ultrasound showed bilateral renal atrophy. The patient underwent temporary catheterization of the right internal jugular vein and received regular blood purification treatment after surgery. After comprehensive evaluation of the patient's condition, a diagnosis of chronic kidney disease with stage 5 was made, for which long-term renal replacement therapy was needed. In January 2021, he underwent surgery for a left forearm arteriovenous fistula. Regular blood dialysis was performed after surgery, assisted by symptomatic supportive treatments to promote hematopoiesis, control his blood pressure and uric acid, and regulate his calcium and phosphorus metabolism.

The patient underwent hemodialysis treatments three times weekly through left forearm arteriovenous fistula, but his anemia was not well corrected. This patient had previously received treatment with 10,000 IU of erythropoietin at QW and later

L. Chen (✉) · W.-X. Chang (✉)
Tianjin First Central Hospital, Tianjin, China

© The Author(s) 2025
B.-C. Liu (ed.), *Treatment of Refractory Renal Anemia*,
https://doi.org/10.1007/978-981-97-7636-8_13

77

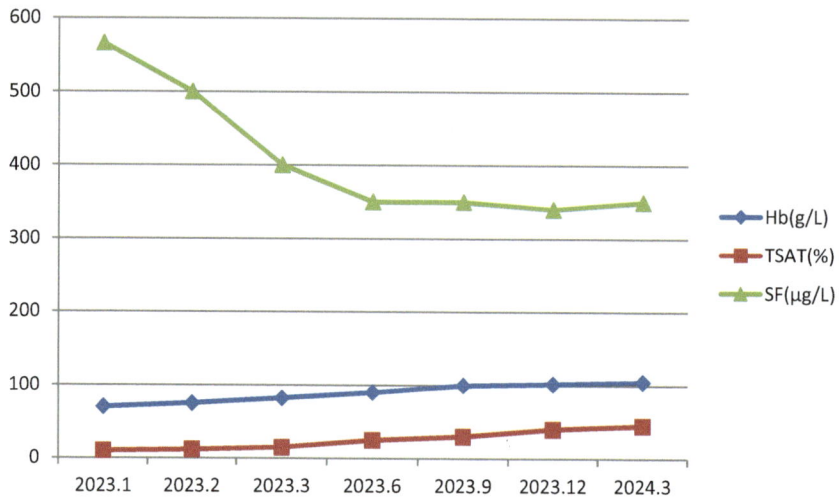

Fig. 13.1 Changes in hemoglobin (Hb), transferrin saturation (TAST), and serum ferritin (SF) levels

transitioned to 10,000 IU of BIW, but his hemoglobin still fluctuated around 70 to 80 g/L.

The patient received a series of laboratory experiments to determine the potential causes for his ESA hyporesponsiveness, including antinuclear antibody series, vasculitis and whether there were conditions such as cirrhosis and splenomegaly, adequacy of dialysis, and so on. His URR is 65% and Kt/V is 1.5. The parathyroid hormone is 300 pg/ml. Abdominal CT scan shows no clear manifestation of cirrhosis and splenomegaly. The patient's liver function showed no abnormalities, with ALT levels of 15.1 U/L, AST 25.7 U/L，and TBIL 7.74 μmol/L. At the same time, no special abnormalities were observed in other secondary factors. His serum iron, total iron-binding capacity, and transferrin saturation were low, but ferritin was high. He was assumed to have an iron metabolism disorder, a microinflammatory state, and erythropoietin resistance. We then prescribed him roxadustat 100 mg thrice weekly; he had a gradual increase in hemoglobin to 90 g/L; we then raised his dosage of roxadustat to 150 mg TIW after 1 month considering his body weight. We could see the gradual increase of his hemoglobin to a stable target level. His iron metabolism significantly improved compared to before, with an increase in serum iron and transferrin saturation, a decrease in ferritin, and an increase in iron utilization (Fig. 13.1).

13.2 Discussion

Although renal anemia has attracted widespread attention from clinicians, many chronic kidney disease patients still have concomitant renal anemia with low hemoglobin [1–3]. The causes of anemia in chronic kidney disease patients are multifaceted and can include erythropoietin deficiency, abnormal iron metabolism, blood loss, chronic inflammation, shortened red blood cell survival time, infection, oxidative stress, and nutritional deficiency [4–6]. Growing evidence suggests that excessive levels of ferritin can explain the causes of iron metabolism disorders in many patients with chronic kidney disease [7]. Iron is a central regulatory factor responsible for maintaining systemic iron homeostasis. As the only known exporter of iron to the plasma, ferritin can maintain systemic iron balance by regulating membrane iron transporters on the surface of intestinal cells, liver cells, macrophages, and placental cells [8]. Iron-regulatory factors are themselves regulated by various mechanisms, such as chronic inflammation, iron metabolism, hypoxia, and demand for red blood cell generation. The most typical mechanism is that liver ferritin is directly transcriptionally activated through the signal transduction and activator of transcription 3 (STAT3) signaling pathway in the inflammatory microenvironment, especially through the inflammatory cytokines interleukin (IL-6) and IL-1β [9]. In fact, many patients with chronic kidney disease have a chronic inflammatory state [10]. Chronic inflammation is particularly prominent in patients with maintenance hemodialysis combined with viral hepatitis, leading to an increase in ferritin, which hinders iron metabolism and, in turn, makes iron absorption difficult [6]. Ferritin plays a crucial role in iron metabolism and renal anemia, and regulating ferritin has become a new treatment strategy for renal anemia [11].

At present, the application of erythropoietin and iron supplementation are the cornerstones for treating renal anemia, but many concerns remain. On the one hand, several studies on erythropoietin have shown that it does not significantly improve the prognosis of chronic kidney disease but instead increases cardiovascular events and mortality [12, 13]. On the other hand, much evidence suggests a close relationship between unstable iron and oxidative stress, bacterial growth, severe gastrointestinal side effects, and hypersensitivity, increasing the risk of infection and mortality, especially in patients with chronic kidney disease who receive intravenous iron supplementation [14, 15]. A randomized controlled trial found that intravenous iron brought serious side effects, including cardiovascular and infectious diseases [16]. Therefore, many other methods have been explored for treating renal anemia. The clinical application of the low-oxygen inducible factor proline enhancer enzyme inhibitor roxadustat provides a new opportunity for the treatment of refractory renal anemia [17, 18]. The mechanism of action of roxadustat involves multiple processes, including regulating iron metabolism to inhibit the generation of ferritin, regulating endogenous erythropoietin gene expression and expression of its receptor, promoting the release of reserve ferritin, and improving the inflammatory status of patients with chronic kidney disease. Through the abovementioned mechanisms, it can achieve the multitarget treatment of renal anemia.

This study reported a special case of maintenance hemodialysis anemia complicated with viral hepatitis. This patient was diagnosed with chronic hepatitis B virus infection, but no special abnormalities were noted in the liver function, and there were no complications such as cirrhosis, splenomegaly, portal hypertension, and so on. His nutritional status was good. According to the literature, patients with viral hepatitis are in a chronic inflammatory state, and their ferritin metabolism is disrupted, which then increases the difficulty of treatment once renal anemia occurs [19]. In this present case, the use of a large amount of erythropoietin for a long time did not improve his hemoglobin. After adjusting to roxadustat, his anemia was corrected with iron metabolism improved. Meanwhile, his hypersensitive CRP decreased, and the level of ferritin decreased as well.

References

1. Ma JZ, Ebben J, Xia H, Collins AJ. Hematocrit level and associated mortality in hemodialysis patients. J Am Soc Nephrol. 1999;10(3):610–9.
2. Xia H, Ebben J, Ma JZ, Collins AJ. Hematocrit levels and hospitalization risks in hemodialysis patients. J Am Soc Nephrol. 1999;10(6):1309–16.
3. Stauffer ME, Fan T. Prevalence of anemia in chronic kidney disease in the United States. PLoS One. 2014;9(1):e84943.
4. Weiss G, Ganz T, Goodnough LT. Anemia of inflammation. Blood. 2019;133(1):40–50.
5. Babitt JL, Lin HY. Mechanisms of anemia in CKD. J Am Soc Nephrol. 2012;23(10):1631–4.
6. Fishbane S, Spinowitz B. Update on anemia in ESRD and earlier stages of CKD: core curriculum 2018. Am J Kidney Dis. 2018;71(3):423–35.
7. Ueda N, Takasawa K. Role of hepcidin-25 in chronic kidney disease: anemia and beyond. Curr Med Chem. 2017;24(14):1417–52.
8. Nemeth E, Tuttle MS, Powelson J, et al. Hepcidin regulates cellular iron efflux by binding to ferroportin and inducing its internalization. Science. 2004;306(5704):2090–3.
9. Pietrangelo A, Dierssen U, Valli L, et al. STAT3 is required for IL-6-gp130-dependent activation of hepcidin in vivo. Gastroenterology. 2007;132(1):294–300.
10. Akchurin OM, Kaskel F. Update on inflammation in chronic kidney disease. Blood Purif. 2015;39(1–3):84–92.
11. Malyszko J, Malyszko JS, Matuszkiewicz-Rowinska J. Hepcidin as a therapeutic target for anemia and inflammation associated with chronic kidney disease. Expert Opin Ther Targets. 2019;23(5):407–21.
12. Solomon SD, Uno H, Lewis EF, et al. Erythropoietic response and outcomes in kidney disease and type 2 diabetes. N Engl J Med. 2010;363(12):1146–55.
13. Koulouridis I, Alfayez M, Trikalinos TA, Balk EM, Jaber BL. Dose of erythropoiesis-stimulating agents and adverse outcomes in CKD: a metaregression analysis. Am J Kidney Dis. 2013;61(1):44–56.
14. Li X, Cole SR, Kshirsagar AV, Fine JP, Stürmer T, Brookhart MA. Safety of dynamic intravenous iron administration strategies in hemodialysis patients. Clin J Am Soc Nephrol. 2019;14(5):728–37.
15. Bailie GR, Larkina M, Goodkin DA, et al. Data from the dialysis outcomes and practice patterns study validate an association between high intravenous iron doses and mortality. Kidney Int. 2015;87(1):162–8.
16. Agarwal R, Kusek JW, Pappas MK. A randomized trial of intravenous and oral iron in chronic kidney disease. Kidney Int. 2015;88(4):905–14.
17. Koury MJ, Haase VH. Anaemia in kidney disease: harnessing hypoxia responses for therapy. Nat Rev Nephrol. 2015;11(7):394–410.
18. Bonomini M, del Vecchio L, Sirolli V, Locatelli F. New treatment approaches for the anemia of CKD. Am J Kidney Dis. 2016;67(1):133–42.
19. Nagashima M, Kudo M, Chung H, et al. Regulatory failure of serum prohepcidin levels in patients with hepatitis C. Hepatol Res. 2006;36(4):288–93.

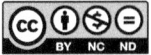

The Role of Intravenous Iron Supplementation in the Treatment of Renal Anemia with Roxadustat

Mu-Yao Ye, Ying-Hong Liu, Hong Liu, and Xiao Fu

14.1 Case Presentation

The patient was a 63-year-old male who was hospitalized for hyperglycemia for 12 years and edema and high creatinine for 5 years, which then aggravated for 1 month. The patient was diagnosed with type 2 diabetes 12 years earlier due to polydipsia and polyuria. Five years ago, he went to the hospital due to edema of both lower limbs. His blood pressure was 155/95 mmHg, urinary protein 2+, and creatinine about 200 μmol/L. The patient was diagnosed with type 2 diabetes, diabetic nephropathy (stage G3A3), and renal hypertension. Insulin was administered to control blood glucose; diuretics were used to reduce swelling, and antihypertensive drugs and kidney protection drugs were simultaneously used. After treatment, the patient's edema was attenuated. In the past 5 years, edema has occurred repeatedly, mainly in both lower limbs, with a concave appearance. The edema was mild in the morning and severe in the evening, with occasional swelling of the eyelids. Repeated re-examinations revealed fluctuations in the urine protein concentration ranging from + to 3+, and serum creatinine gradually increased. Six months earlier, serum creatinine reached 527 μmol/L. One month earlier, the edema gradually worsened, and the urine volume gradually decreased to around 600–800 mL per day. His urine volume reached approximately 1000 mL when taking tolazamide. After medication, the patient's edema gradually worsened, and he developed shortness of breath after exercise, requiring a high pillow position at night. The patient had a poor appetite and occasional nausea, but no vomiting.

Laboratory examination showed the following: Hb, 72 g/L; blood urea nitrogen, 17.8 mmol/L; creatinine, 723 μmol/L; and albumin, 34 g/L. The iron metabolism index showed that ferritin was 96.1 ng/mL; serum iron was 5.9 μmol/L, and

M.-Y. Ye · Y.-H. Liu · H. Liu · X. Fu (✉)
Department of Nephrology, The Second Xiangya Hospital of Central South University, Changsha, China
e-mail: fuxiao2064@csu.edu.cn

© The Author(s) 2025
B.-C. Liu (ed.), *Treatment of Refractory Renal Anemia*,
https://doi.org/10.1007/978-981-97-7636-8_14

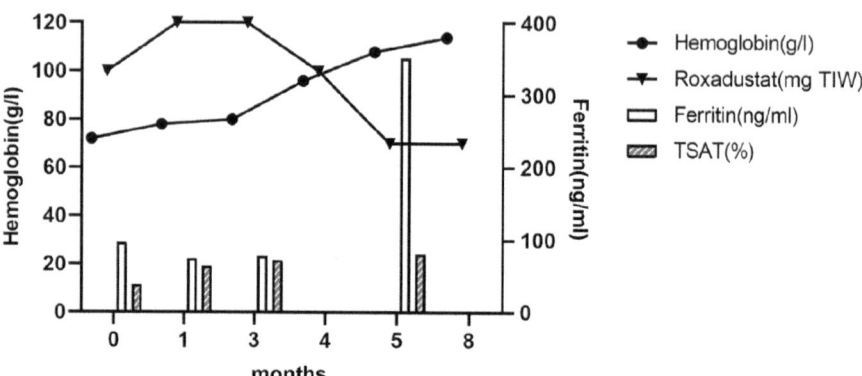

Fig. 14.1 Changes in hemoglobin levels, roxadustat dosage, and ferritin and TSAT levels

transferrin saturation (TSAT) was 11.3%. The patient accepted peritoneal dialysis treatment. The plan was to keep three bags of 1.5% peritoneal dialysis solution (2 L) for 4 hours during the day and one bag of 1.5% peritoneal dialysis solution (2 L) in the abdomen for 12 hours at night. Oral roxadustat 100 mg TIW and oral iron 200 mg QD were given to treat renal anemia.

One month later, Hb reached 78 g/L, but ferritin decreased to 74.2 ng/mL, with a TSAT of 19.1%. The peritoneal equilibration test showed a total KT/V of 1.57, a total Ccr of 57.14, and a high average transport score of 0.78. The peritoneal dialysis was deemed adequate. Therefore, roxadustat was administered at a dose of 120 mg of TIW, and oral iron supplementation was continued.

In the third month, Hb stabilized at 80 g/L; ferritin was 78.1 ng/mL, and TSAT was 21.7%. The body composition analyzer showed that the patient's target weight was 58 kg. The rate of increase in Hb remained substandard, and intravenous (IV) iron supplementation treatment should be attempted. IV iron (100 mg BIW) was administered for 4 weeks, with a total of 800 mg iron supplementation. The patient still took 120 mg roxadustat TIW. In the fourth month, the Hb concentration reached 96 g/L, and oral iron supplementation was administered. The roxadustat dose was reduced to 100 mg TIW. In the fifth month, Hb was 108 g/L; ferritin was 351.6 ng/mL, and TSAT was 24.3%. Roxadustat was further reduced to 70 mg TIW along with oral iron. The Hb concentration in the eighth month was 114 g/L, and the drug dosage remained unchanged. Figure 14.1 shows the changes in Hb levels, roxadustat dosage, and ferritin and transferrin saturation levels.

14.2   Discussion

Renal anemia is one of the major problems faced by dialysis patients with chronic kidney disease (CKD). How to treat renal anemia is also a problem that nephrologists are trying to solve. Due to the insufficiency of erythropoietin (EPO) in patients with renal anemia, we focused on supplementation with EPO, such as recombinant human erythropoietin (rhuEPO), which is used to supplement EPO externally, and roxadustat, the HIF-PHI that promotes the production of endogenous EPO. Because of the convenience of its oral dosage, roxadustat has gradually become widely used in CKD patients who are not receiving dialysis or peritoneal dialysis. The pharmacological mechanisms of roxadustat are diverse; roxadustat not only promotes the generation of endogenous EPO and upregulates EPO receptors but also regulates iron metabolism. Roxadustat can also upregulate DMT1 and increase intestinal iron absorption [1], so it is widely believed that oral iron supplements can meet these needs. It can also upregulate the expression of transferrin and transferrin receptor, so as to increase iron uptake by proerythrocytes [2]. It does not directly affect the synthesis of hepcidin but induces a decrease in the serum hepcidin level by affecting iron metabolism. In addition, some studies have shown that Hb synthesis is maintained with decreased TSAT and serum ferritin during roxadustat therapy when the ferritin concentration is lower than 100 mg/mL [3]. Therefore, roxadustat claims that IV iron is unnecessary when it is used for the treatment of renal anemia. That statement has been written into the medication package insert.

In this patient, Hb increased by only 6 g/L, but ferritin decreased in the first month of roxadustat treatment. Hb, ferritin, and TSAT did not obviously change from the first to the third month. Patients with other factors that may cause bleeding or hematopoietic disorders were excluded. Since the patient's ferritin level had always been in a state of absolute iron deficiency (ferritin <100 ng/mL), although TSAT increased to more than 20%, as the rate of increase in Hb did not reach the standard, we still considered that oral iron supplementation was ineffective. Possible reasons for this patient include insufficient iron intake caused by poor appetite and iron absorption disorders caused by gastrointestinal dysfunction. Therefore, we tried IV iron supplementation. After IV iron supplementation at 800 mg, the ferritin level significantly improved. The Hb concentration also improved, with the monthly increase rate reaching the standard. After sufficient iron supplementation, the dosage of roxadustat was gradually decreased to a maintenance level. Figure 14.1 shows that the increase in hemoglobin was not related to the dose of roxadustat but was closely related to the level of ferritin.

We reviewed the literature and found that clinical studies have suggested that, compared with rhuEPO in dialysis patients, roxadustat increases serum iron, transferrin, and total iron-binding capacity, while the TSAT and ferritin levels decrease slightly, and the level of hepcidin decreases significantly [4, 5]. Oral or IV iron supplementation generally results in increases in TSAT and ferritin. In clinical trials of roxadustat and rhuEPO, patients were encouraged to take oral iron as the first-line iron supplement, with no specific dose or frequency requirements. Parenteral iron was withheld except as rescue therapy [6]. Although oral iron supplementation is advocated in the instruction manual of roxadustat, IV iron was allowed in clinical trials if the patient's Hb did not respond adequately, and the patient was considered iron-deficient. Treatment with drugs continued during IV iron administration, and the iron supplement was started orally once the patient was iron-replete, which was defined as ferritin ≥100 ng/mL and TSAT ≥20% [7]. As intravenous iron supplementation might increase the risk of allergic reactions, inflammation, iron overload, and cardiovascular morbidity, a number of guidelines limit and strictly guide its prescription [8].

Therefore, this does not mean that patients who use roxadustat cannot receive IV iron supplementation. In clinical practice, patients have many individual differences. When oral iron supplementation cannot meet the patient's hematopoietic raw material needs, IV iron should be supplemented in a timely manner. Although oral iron supplementation can increase the patient's iron reserve, roxadustat promotes hematopoiesis and the consumption of iron. The amount of iron stored in the body varies among patients. In the abovementioned clinical trials, the Hb of patients increased, while ferritin and TSAT decreased [5]. On the other hand, it was also confirmed that roxadustat can promote the utilization of iron, but this may cause further iron deficiency in patients. In this case, we initially increased the dose of roxadustat while taking oral iron supplements. However, clinical results have shown that increasing the dose of roxadustat in iron-deficient patients does not effectively improve Hb levels. At the same time, it is necessary to pay attention to the target weight of patients in clinical practice. Due to his edema, the current patient initially weighed more than 60 kg, so we increased his dosage of roxadustat. However, the body composition analyzer showed a target weight of 58 kg, which did not require a dose of 120 mg. This may be one of the reasons why the increase in the dose of roxadustat did not have a significant effect. However, overall, the patient achieved a good outcome. In the end, the Hb level was maintained with a moderate dose of roxadustat.

14.3   Conclusion

In this case, we gained a new understanding of the role of roxadustat in correcting renal anemia. When the improvement in renal anemia does not meet the standard, in addition to seeking other reasons, clinicians should not simply increase the dosage of roxadustat. More attention needs to be paid to the iron metabolism of patients. Although oral iron supplementation is sufficient for most patients, if ferritin and hemoglobin do not obviously improve in patients receiving oral iron supplementation, intravenous iron supplementation is needed, and they should be monitored for the long term.

References

1. Yang L, Wang D, Wang XT, Lu YP, Zhu L. The roles of hypoxia-inducible Factor-1 and iron regulatory protein 1 in iron uptake induced by acute hypoxia. Biochem Biophys Res Commun. 2018;507(1–4):128–35.
2. Li M, Tang X, Liao Z, et al. Hypoxia and low temperature upregulate transferrin to induce hypercoagulability at high altitude. Blood. 2022;140(19):2063–75.
3. Ogawa C, Tsuchiya K, Tomosugi N, Maeda K. Hypoxia-inducible factor prolyl hydroxylase domain inhibitor may maintain hemoglobin synthesis at lower serum ferritin and transferrin saturation levels than darbepoetin alfa. PLoS One. 2021;16(6):e0252439.

4. Chen N, Hao C, Liu BC, et al. Roxadustat treatment for anemia in patients undergoing long-term dialysis. N Engl J Med. 2019;381(11):1011–22.
5. Charytan C, Manllo-Karim R, Martin ER, et al. A randomized trial of roxadustat in anemia of kidney failure: SIERRAS study. Kidney Int Rep. 2021;6(7):1829–39.
6. Pergola PE, Charytan C, Little DJ, et al. Changes in iron availability with roxadustat in nondialysis- and dialysis-dependent patients with anemia of CKD. Kidney360. 2022;3(9):1511–28.
7. Provenzano R, Shutov E, Eremeeva L, et al. Roxadustat for anemia in patients with end-stage renal disease incident to dialysis. Nephrol Dial Transplant. 2021;36(9):1717–30.
8. Kassianides X, Hazara AM, Bhandari S. Improving the safety of intravenous iron treatments for patients with chronic kidney disease. Expert Opin Drug Saf. 2020;20(1):23–35.

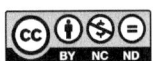

Roxadustat for Anemia in a Patient with Chronic Kidney Disease Not Receiving Dialysis

15

Panai Song and Lin Sun

15.1 Case Presentation

A 66-year-old female was given oral metformin and gliclazide and later switched to linagliptin management when a diagnosis of type 2 diabetes was made because of high blood glucose 17 years ago. Four years earlier, a diagnosis of diabetic nephropathy (stage III) was made with elevated serum creatinine (approximately 100 μmol/L), but this was not emphasized. One year ago, her serum creatinine gradually increased to 400 μmol/L, and she was initially treated with Shen-Shuai-Ning capsules. One month ago, after contracting COVID-19, she complained of chest distress, palpitations, and fatigue, with a serum creatinine concentration of 650 μmol/L and a hemoglobin concentration of 69 g/L. Her symptoms did not improve significantly after she received antihyperglycemic, antihypertensive, or antihyperlipidemic agents at the local hospital, so she came to our hospital for further treatment.

She had a history of hypertension for 17 years and was regularly taking antihypertensive drugs (amlodipine tablets). She also had a history of ureterolithotomy 20 years ago. No other specific information on personal or family history was found. Her blood pressure was 160/64 mmHg, and her body weight was 50 kg. Physical examination suggested a severe anemic face and mild concave edema in both lower extremities.

Laboratory examinations revealed the following: WBC, 7.9×10^9/L; RBC, 3.32×10^{12}/L, hemoglobin concentration, 69 g/L; platelet count, 258×10^9/L;

P. Song · L. Sun (✉)
Department of Nephrology, The Second Xiangya Hospital, Central South University, Changsha, China

Hunan Key Laboratory of Kidney Disease and Blood Purification, Changsha, Hunan, China

© The Author(s) 2025
B.-C. Liu (ed.), *Treatment of Refractory Renal Anemia*,
https://doi.org/10.1007/978-981-97-7636-8_15

hematocrit (HCT), 23.7%; mean corpuscular volume (MCV), 71.4 fl; mean corpuscular hemoglobin (MVH), 20.8 pg; mean corpuscular-hemoglobin concentration (MCHC), 291 g/L; C-reactive protein concentration, 1.89 mg/L; serum
total protein concentration, 57.1 g/L; albumin concentration, 36.3 g/L; blood
urea nitrogen concentration, 29.9 mmol/L; creatinine concentration, 626 μmol/L
(ref 44–133 μmol/L); uric acid concentration, 586 μmol/L; serum calcium concentration, 1.82 mmol/L; and phosphorus concentration, 1.67 mmol/L. Serology
for autoantibodies (including anti-nuclear, anti-double-stranded DNA, anti-glomerular basement membrane, and anti-neutrophilic cytoplasmic antibodies) and
for viral infections (hepatitis B and C or HIV infections) were all negative.
Moreover, there was no evidence of hematological disease according to serum
protein electrophoresis or immunofixation electrophoresis. Ultrasonography of
the abdomen revealed a cholecystic polypus. Cardiac ultrasonography revealed
that the left atrium was slightly enlarged and that the left ventricular wall was
thickened. In addition, her nutritional status was good, and her intact parathyroid hormone was 209 pg/mL. In addition, a biomarker of stored iron was
detected (ferritin 124 ng/mL). The ferritin level indicated that she had functional iron deficiency.

For treatment, roxadustat at a dose of 100 mg thrice a week with strict control of
blood glucose, blood pressure, and blood lipids was administered. Oral iron supplementation was also given to correct anemia. Her hemoglobin increased gradually to
105 g/L after 1 month. Then, we reduced the dose of roxadustat to 50 mg thrice a
week. During the 3-month follow-up, the patient's hemoglobin stayed at approximately 110 g/L with the same dose of roxadustat (Fig. 15.1). However, the patient's
ferritin levels decreased significantly. Therefore, in the fourth month, her oral iron
was switched to intravenous iron infusion at a dose of 100 mg twice a week, and
1 week later, her ferritin was elevated (Fig. 15.2). The patient's serum creatinine
decreased (from 626 to 461 μmol/L) (Fig. 15.3).

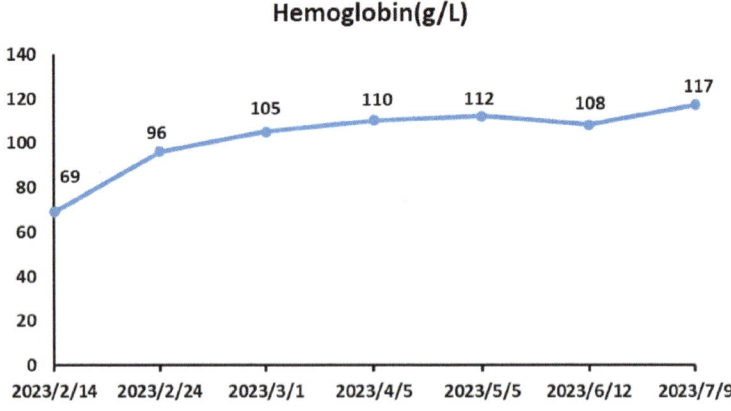

Fig. 15.1 Changes in hemoglobin levels

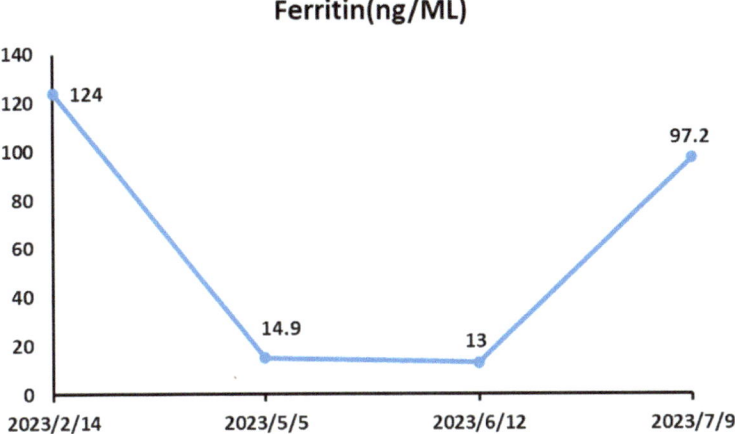

Fig. 15.2 Changes in ferritin levels

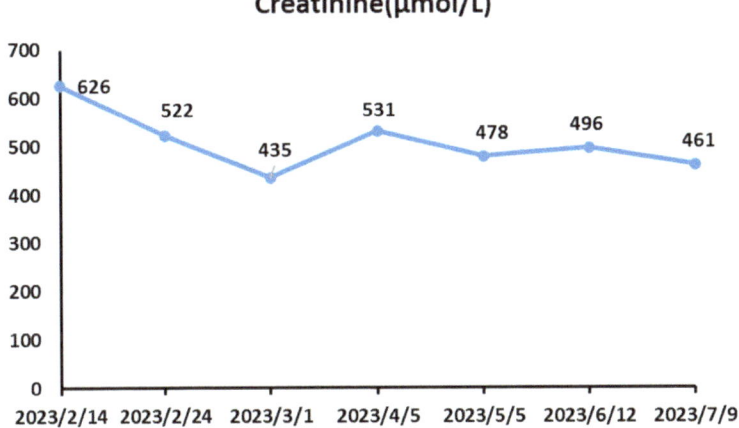

Fig. 15.3 Changes in creatinine levels

15.2   Discussion

An elderly female presented with moderate anemia associated with chronic kidney disease and who was not undergoing dialysis and had a history of type 2 diabetes and hypertension. Before hospitalization, she had not undergone any treatment to correct her anemia. During hospitalization, we used roxadustat and oral iron to correct her anemia. Fortunately, after the beginning of treatment, the patient's anemia significantly improved; her hemoglobin increased from 69 g/L to 105 g/L. Creatinine also dropped from 622 µmol/L to 435 µmol/L. After 4 months of follow-up, the patient's hemoglobin (approximately 110 g/L) and renal function were relatively stable (serum creatinine 400–500 µmol/L).

As a new generation of drugs for renal anemia with novel mechanisms, roxadustat is a first-in-class oral hypoxia-inducible factor (HIF) prolyl hydroxylase inhibitor (PHI) approved for anemia treatment in dialysis-dependent (DD) and nondialysis-dependent (NDD) CKD patients in China, Japan, South Korea, Chile, the European Union, the United Kingdom, and other countries. Through the reversible inhibition of HIF-PH, roxadustat stimulates an erythropoietic response that includes an increase in plasma-endogenous erythropoietin levels, regulation of iron transporter proteins, and a reduction of hepcidin. These effects result in improved iron bioavailability, increased Hb production, and increased red cell mass [1–3]. This patient was initially treated with roxadustat and oral iron to correct anemia, and after 1 month, her hemoglobin level was effectively increased and maintained during follow-up. However, the patient's ferritin did not increase but instead decreased significantly, suggesting that roxadustat may promote iron utilization and decrease iron stores [4].

Previous studies in patients with chronic kidney disease who were not on dialysis have also shown that roxadustat corrected anemia and maintained hemoglobin levels despite lower transferrin saturation and a progressive reduction in ferritin levels with oral iron at moderate doses [3, 5, 6]. This may be related to the fact that roxadustat reduces hepcidin levels, which then promotes intestinal iron absorption and improves iron release from macrophages to transferrin [7]. Therefore, even though we did not measure serum iron, transferrin, or total iron-binding capacity, we can be sure that roxadustat increased iron utilization by increasing hemoglobin in this patient.

Anemia is an independent risk factor for the progression of kidney function in middle-aged and elderly individuals. Attentive management and intervention strategies targeting anemia could reduce the risk of kidney failure and improve the prognosis of the general population [8]. Roxadustat effectively and safely improved renal anemia and delayed the decline in residual renal function (RRF) in patients who developed new PD. [9] In this patient, serum creatinine decreased as the anemia was corrected, and renal function was maintained during the next 4 months of treatment, indicating that the correction of anemia could delay the progression of kidney disease.

Here, we report the case of an anemic patient with chronic kidney disease who was not undergoing dialysis and who had a history of type 2 diabetes and hypertension. Despite the presence of functional iron deficiency in this patient, roxadustat was highly effective at correcting anemia, further confirming that it can improve iron absorption and utilization. In addition, roxadustat may delay the progression of kidney disease by correcting anemia .

References

1. Gupta N, Wish JB. Hypoxia-inducible factor prolyl hydroxylase inhibitors: a potential new treatment for anemia in patients with CKD. Am J Kidney Dis. 2017;69(6):815–26.
2. Barratt J, Andric B, Tataradze A, et al. Roxadustat for the treatment of anaemia in chronic kidney disease patients not on dialysis: a Phase 3, randomized, open-label, active-controlled study (DOLOMITES). Nephrol Dial Transplant. 2021;36(9):1616–28.

3. Chen N, Hao C, Peng X, et al. Roxadustat for anemia in patients with kidney disease not receiving dialysis. N Engl J Med. 2019;381(11):1001–10.
4. Liu J, Zhang A, Hayden JC, et al. Roxadustat (FG-4592) treatment for anemia in dialysis-dependent (DD) and not dialysis-dependent (NDD) chronic kidney disease patients: a systematic review and meta-analysis. Pharmacol Res. 2020;155:104747.
5. Chen N, Qian J, Chen J, et al. Phase 2 studies of oral hypoxia-inducible factor prolyl hydroxylase inhibitor FG-4592 for treatment of anemia in China. Nephrol Dial Transplant. 2017;32(8):1373–86.
6. Provenzano R, Besarab A, Sun CH, et al. Oral hypoxia-inducible factor prolyl hydroxylase inhibitor roxadustat (FG-4592) for the treatment of anemia in patients with CKD. Clin J Am Soc Nephrol. 2016;11(6):982–91.
7. Ganz T, Nemeth E. Hepcidin and iron homeostasis. Biochim Biophys Acta. 2012;1823(9):1434–43.
8. Yang C, Meng Q, Wang H, et al. Anemia and kidney function decline among the middle-aged and elderly in China: a population-based national longitudinal study. Biomed Res Int. 2020;2020:2303541.
9. Wu T, Qi Y, Ma S, et al. Efficacy of Roxadustat on anemia and residual renal function in patients new to peritoneal dialysis. Ren Fail. 2022;44(1):529–40.

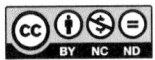

Pure red cell aplasia (PRCA) is a heterogeneous syndrome characterized by isolated red blood cell hematopoietic disorders in the bone marrow without significant involvement of the granulocyte and megakaryocyte series. Pure red cell aplasia is a rare disease caused mainly by genetic mutations, immune abnormalities, viral infections, drugs, antibodies against recombinant human erythropoietin, pregnancy, and hematopoietic stem cell transplantation. Although this disease is relatively rare in patients with CKD and renal anemia, its treatment is often very difficult. Patients develop progressive severe anemia, which severely affects cardiovascular function and quality of life, and can only rely on blood transfusion or immunosuppressive therapy. However, the treatment efficacy is often uncertain, and the prognosis is poor. In this part, several cases of renal anemia complicated with pure red cell aplasia are provided, and new therapies are explored.

Anti-Erythropoietin Antibody-Mediated Pure Red Cell Aplasia

Jiayi Lv and Zhiguo Mao

16.1 Case Presentation

A 78-year-old Chinese man was admitted to the hospital because of dizziness. He was diagnosed with end-stage renal disease due to chronic glomerulonephritis (renal biopsy was not available) and started maintenance hemodialysis three times a week at a local hospital since April 2017. He then received intravenous recombinant human erythropoietin (rHuEPO) at a dose of 3000 U three times per week for anemia treatment. During this time, he received adequate dialysis, and the follow-up results were quite satisfactory. However, in November 2018, his hemoglobin level decreased to 82 g/L, and his rHuEPO dosage was then increased to 5000 U three times per week. Six months later, his hemoglobin level still decreased to 50 g/L. Despite a red blood cell suspension transfusion and rHuEPO treatment, his anemia did not resolve. To determine the cause of anemia, he underwent bone marrow biopsy in June 2019, and a diagnosis of pure red cell aplasia (PRCA) was confirmed. Anti-EPO antibody testing was also performed, and the result was positive, supporting a diagnosis of rHuEPO-mediated PRCA (EPO-PRCA). After the diagnosis, rHuEPO was discontinued, and 0.5 mg/kg/d methylprednisolone, 20 g γ-globulin, and 0.2 g CTX were prescribed. After discharge, the dose of methylprednisolone was gradually reduced to 25 mg/d. In August 2019, syncope occurred because of severe anemia, and his hemoglobin level decreased to 52 g/L. After symptomatic treatment, such as blood transfusion at a local hospital, the patient was admitted to our hospital in September 2019.

He had a 20-year history of hypertension, with a maximum blood pressure of 200/100 mmHg. Antihypertensive drugs (nifedipine controlled-release tablets 30 mg twice a day and valsartan capsules 80 mg once a day) were taken regularly for blood pressure control. The patient denied any history of diabetes, coronary

J. Lv · Z. Mao (✉)
Kidney Institute of CPLA, Department of Nephrology, Changzheng Hospital, Second Military Medical University, Shanghai, China

heart disease, tuberculosis, or viral hepatitis. Diagnoses of thymoma, autoimmune disease, lymphoproliferative disorders, or B19 parvovirus infection were ruled out. The patient also denied exposure to drugs such as phenytoin, azathioprine, or isoniazid. His blood pressure was 200/92 mmHg, and his body weight was 65 kg. Physical examination revealed a pale face and an enlarged cardiac boundary, with no pitting edema in either lower extremity.

Laboratory examination revealed the following: white blood cell (WBC) count, 9.3×10^9/L; red blood cell (RBC) count, 2.36×10^{12}/L; hemoglobin, 71 g/L; mean corpuscular volume, 89.4 fL; mean corpuscular hemoglobin, 30.1 pg; reticulocyte count, 22.2×10^9/L; C-reactive protein, 3.52 mg/L; erythrocyte sedimentation rate, 85 mm/h; serum total protein, 63.7 g/L; albumin, 32.4 g/L; blood urea nitrogen, 35.7 mmol/L; creatinine, 842 μmol/L (reference range, 57–111 μmol/L); serum calcium, 2.06 mmol/L; phosphorus, 1.80 mmol/L; potassium, 7 mmol/L; uric acid, 336 μmol/L; parathormone, 209.5 pg/mL; carcinoembryonic antigen, 6.45 μg/L; and CA125, 35.42 U/mL. Other serological test results for tumor markers, autoantibodies (including anti-nuclear, anti-double-stranded DNA, anti-glomerular basement membrane, and anti-neutrophil cytoplasmic antibodies) and viral infections (hepatitis B and C or HIV infections) were all negative. Serum protein electrophoresis, immunofixation electrophoresis, and Coombs tests were also negative.

We also evaluated biomarkers of iron status, including stored iron and functional iron, and the results were as follows: ferritin, >2000 μg/L; serum iron, 25.5 μmol/L; total iron-binding capacity, 33.1 μmol/L; and transferrin saturation, 77%. In addition, the patient's folic acid concentration was greater than 90.6 nmol/L, and his vitamin B12 concentration was 443 pmol/L. We therefore ruled out anemia caused by insufficient hematopoietic raw materials. Bone marrow biopsy and anti-EPO antibody analysis were not repeated because they had already been performed at another hospital, and the patient refused to undergo repeat tests.

For treatment, adequate hemodialysis was performed. Blood pressure was controlled within 150/90 mmHg with nifedipine controlled-release tablets and sacubitril valsartan sodium tablets. For anemia treatment, roxadustat was prescribed at a dosage of 120 mg three times per week. Considering the excessive iron load of the patient, iron treatment was not administered. Moreover, immunosuppressive therapy was also modified. Methylprednisolone was continued at a dose of 25 mg/d. In addition, cyclosporin was prescribed at a dosage of 100 mg twice a day, and the plasma concentration of cyclosporin was monitored to ensure that it ranged between 100 and 200 ng/mL. After 1 month of treatment, the hemoglobin level increased to 108 g/L. However, because of financial problems, roxadustat was discontinued for 2 months, and the patient's hemoglobin level again decreased to 81 g/L. After restarting roxadustat treatment, the hemoglobin level increased to 119 g/L. After 1 month of treatment, we started to decrease the dosage of methylprednisolone. Almost 4 months later, we began to gradually decrease the dose of cyclosporin. Only roxadustat was used for anemia treatment, and during the follow-up period, the patient's hemoglobin level was maintained at a satisfactory level (Fig. 16.1).

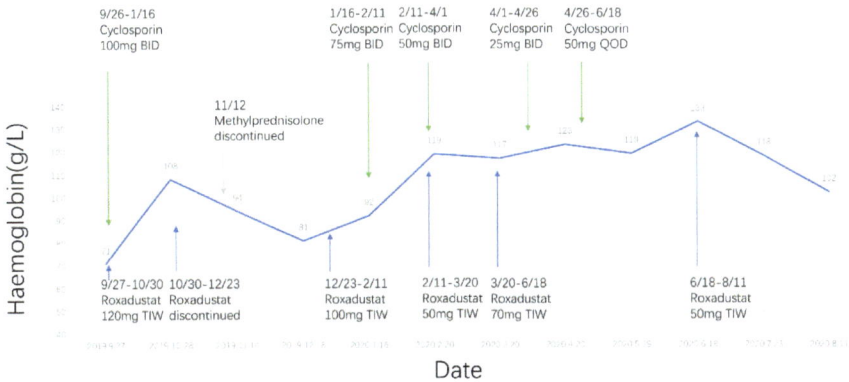

Fig. 16.1 Clinical course of the patient

16.2 Discussion

This elderly male regular hemodialysis patient presented with severe anemia. Previous rHuEPO treatment was effective. However, the patient was hyporesponsive to rHuEPO.

The patient's blood test revealed normocytic normochromic anemia, with a low proportion of reticulocytes and normal WBC and platelet counts. Bone marrow biopsy revealed PRCA. PRCA can be classified as congenital or acquired. Congenital PRCA, such as Diamond–Blackfan anemia, is often caused by genetic mutations [1]. A retrospective European study revealed an incidence of 1.5–5.0 per 10^6 in children younger than 15 years of age [2]. The causes of acquired aplastic anemia are noted to vary. Primary aplastic anemia is mostly caused by autoimmune disorders, whereas secondary aplastic anemia may be secondary to thymoma, infection (especially B19 parvovirus), drugs and chemical poisons, hemolytic anemia, systemic lupus erythematosus, severe malnutrition, malignant tumors, and anti-EPO antibody production [1]. The patient had no history of thymoma; no other blood system-related abnormalities were found by bone marrow biopsy, and he denied a history of exposure to related drugs. In addition, the patient had received rHuEPO for a long time to treat anemia, and the anti-rHuEPO antibody test result was positive; therefore, a diagnosis of EPO-PRCA could be made.

Globally, EPO-PRCA is relatively rare. Since rHuEPO was first used to treat anemia in 1989, only dozens of cases have been reported. The cause of rHuEPO may be related to the genetic background, the type of rHuEPO used, the method of drug delivery, and the duration of administration. Studies have shown that EPO-α is more likely to induce EPO-PRCA than EPO-β, with approximately ten times more cases of EPO-PRCA caused by EPO-α than by EPO-β [3]. In addition, subcutaneous injection of rHuEPO is more likely to induce EPO-PRCA than intravenous administration. The incidence of PRCA caused by subcutaneous injection is 1.6/10000, while the incidence of PRCA caused by intravenous injection is only 0.02/10000 [4]. EPO-PRCA is characterized by progressive, severe, and isolated anemia of sudden onset. The following two criteria must be met for EPO-PRCA diagnosis: a diagnosis of PRCA supported by bone marrow biopsy pathological findings and a positive anti-rHuEPO antibody test result [3]. At present, there are several methods for the detection of anti-rHuEPO antibodies, including radioim-munoprecipitation assays (RIPA), enzyme-linked immunosorbent assays (ELISAs), and surface plasmon resonance methods (BIAcore biosensor immunoassays) [5–7]. Patients with EPO-PRCA also have elevated ferritin and TSAT levels, suggesting that these patients have iron utilization disorders.

For the treatment of EPO-PRCA, mainstream options include immediate ces-sation of rHuEPO, restrictive transfusion of red cell suspensions, and immuno-suppressive therapies [8]. There are also studies showing that kidney transplantation could be a viable option for end-stage renal disease (ESRD) patients with EPO-PRCA. Twelve out of 13 ESRD patients with EPO-PRCA who underwent kidney transplantation have fully recovered [9]. Since the oral hypoxia-inducible factor-prolyl hydroxylase inhibitor roxadustat was developed for anemia treatment, it might be a new option for EPO-PRCA patients. In par-ticular, for patients who have already achieved long-term clinical remission, the reuse of rHuEPO is not recommended; therefore, roxadustat could be an alterna-tive option. Although our patient was prescribed immunosuppressive therapy and roxadustat together for EPO-PRCA treatment, there are a few case reports of roxadustat alone being effective for EPO-PRCA, which would be very promising for EPO-PRCA treatment [10–13]. However, the use of roxadustat in EPO-PRCA treatment remains to be limited; thus, the effectiveness of roxadustat should be further confirmed.

Here, we report the case of an ESRD patient with EPO-PRCA on regular hemo-dialysis. After immunosuppressive and roxadustat treatment, anemia was resolved. Interestingly, because of financial problems, the patient discontinued roxadustat for 2 months, and his hemoglobin levels dropped significantly, which verified the effec-tiveness of roxadustat from another perspective. Therefore, roxadustat is a new option for the treatment of EPO-PRCA [10, 11, 13].

References

1. Gurnari C, Maciejewski JP. How I manage acquired pure red cell aplasia in adults. Blood. 2021;137(15):2001–9.
2. Da Costa L, Leblanc T, Mohandas N. Diamond-blackfan anemia. Blood. 2020;136(11):1262–73.
3. Casadevall N, Cournoyer D, Marsh J, et al. Recommendations on haematological criteria for the diagnosis of epoetin-induced pure red cell aplasia. Eur J Haematol. 2004;73(6):389–96.
4. Locatelli F, Aljama P, Barany P, et al. Erythropoiesis-stimulating agents and antibody-medi-ated pure red-cell aplasia: here are we now and where do we go from here? Nephrol Dial Transplant. 2004;19(2):288–93.
5. Casadevall N, Nataf J, Viron B, et al. Pure red-cell aplasia and antierythropoietin antibodies in patients treated with recombinant erythropoietin. N Engl J Med. 2002;346(7):469–75.
6. Castelli G, Famularo A, Semino C, et al. Detection of anti-erythropoietin antibodies in haemodialysis patients treated with recombinant human-erythropoietin. Pharmacol Res. 2000;41(3):313–8.

7. Swanson SJ. New technologies for the detection of antibodies to therapeutic proteins. Dev Biol (Basel). 2003;112:127–33.

8. Sawada K, Fujishima N, Hirokawa M. Acquired pure red cell aplasia: updated review of treatment. Br J Haematol. 2008;142(4):505–14.

9. Chen XM, Li H, Wu Y, Wang LL, Bai YJ, Shi YY. Case report: dynamic antibody monitoring in a case of anti-recombinant human erythropoietin-mediated pure red cell aplasia with prolonged course after kidney transplantation. Front Immunol. 2022;13:1049444.

10. Li S, Chen X, Hu P, et al. Roxadustat improves erythropoietin antibody-mediated pure red cell aplasia in a patient with hemodialysis. Blood Purif. 2022;51(2):189–92.

11. Wan K, Yin Y, Luo Z, Cheng J. Remarkable response to roxadustat in a case of anti-erythropoietin antibody-mediated pure red cell aplasia. Ann Hematol. 2021;100(2):591–3.

12. Wu Y, Cai X, Ni J, Lin X. Resolution of epoetin-induced pure red cell aplasia, successful rechallenge with roxadustat. Int J Lab Hematol. 2020;42(6):e291–3.

13. Wu R, Peng Y. Roxadustat on anti-erythropoietin antibody-related pure red cell aplasia in the patient with end-stage renal disease. Semin Dial. 2021;34(4):319–22.

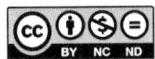

Treatment of Erythropoietin-Induced Pure Red Cell Aplastic Anemia

17

Jia-Feng Liu, Li-Jun Mou, and Kun-Ling Ma

17.1 Case Presentation

A 70-year-old man had repeated instances of foamy urine accompanied by elevated serum creatinine for 5 years before admission and was treated with oral traditional Chinese medicine but with no significant efficacy. He was admitted to our hospital for edema of the lower extremities and puffy eyelids for 4 days.

He had a 9-year history of hypertension and regularly took antihypertensive drugs (telmisartan and amlodipine besylate tablets). He also had a 5-year history of gout, for which he took nonsteroidal anti-inflammatory drugs (NSAIDs) for flares, and he recently took a diclofenac sodium capsule. No other special information was noted in his personal or family history. Physical examination revealed a pale face and moderate pitting edema in both the lower extremities and the eyelids.

Laboratory examinations revealed a hemoglobin level of 68 g/L and a reticulocyte count (%) of 1.58%, while the white blood cell (WBC) count and platelet count were within the normal range. The serum total protein concentration was 56.2 g/L; the serum albumin concentration was 32.6 g/L; the serum potassium concentration was 5.40 mmol/L; the calcium concentration was 1.97 mmol/L, the phosphorus concentration was 2.08 mmol/L; the creatinine concentration was 819 μmol/L; and the uric acid concentration was 539 μmol/L. Urine examination results were as follows: urine protein, 2+; urine microalbumin, 3648.65 mg/g.Cr; urine IgG, 505.41 mg/g.Cr; urine transferrin, 176.22 mg/g.Cr; urine α1 microglobulin, 152.16 mg/g.Cr; and 24-hour urine protein quantification, 3108 mg. The serum iron level was 6.8 μmol/L; the transferrin saturation was 17.1%, and the parathyroid hormone level was 466.10 pg/mL. The results of the serological tests for tumor markers, autoantibodies (including anti-nuclear, anti-double-stranded DNA,

J.-F. Liu (✉) · L.-J. Mou · K.-L. Ma
Department of Nephrology, The Second Affiliated Hospital of Zhejiang University School of Medicine, Hang Zhou City, China
e-mail: jiafengliu21@zju.edu.cn

© The Author(s) 2025
B.-C. Liu (ed.), *Treatment of Refractory Renal Anemia*,
https://doi.org/10.1007/978-981-97-7636-8_17

anti-glomerular basement membrane, and anti-neutrophilic cytoplasmic antibodies) and viral infections (hepatitis B and C or HIV infections) were all negative. Moreover, there was no evidence of hematological disease (serum protein electrophoresis or immunofixation electrophoresis) or hemolytic disease (Coombs test, CD55, and CD59 expression). Ultrasonography of the abdomen revealed shrinkage of both kidneys (left kidney size, 8.59 × 4.52 cm; right kidney size, 7.84 × 3.85 cm), regular kidney morphology, a smooth kidney envelope, and an enhanced parenchymal echo.

Therefore, the patient was diagnosed with chronic kidney disease (stage 5), renal anemia, hyperphosphatemia, hypocalcemia, secondary hyperparathyroidism, hypertension, and gout.

He was initially treated with intravenous recombinant human erythropoietin (Yibiao) at a dosage of 10,000 U once a week combined with iron supplementation on March 23, 2020 for treating anemia. Febuxostat was given to treat gout; carvedilol and nifedipine were given to control blood pressure; Shenshuaining capsules, compound α-ketoacid tablets, and Bailing capsules were given to protect the kidneys; and sevelamer carbonate was given to reduce phosphorus. Temporary hemodialysis was followed by peritoneal dialysis catheterization and daily peritoneal dialysis treatment. During the follow-up from May 2020 to October 2020, the patient's hemoglobin levels were maintained at 104–107 g/L. However, his hemoglobin level decreased to 56 g/L on January 6, 2021, and he was hospitalized again.

Laboratory examinations revealed a hemoglobin level of 47 g/L and a reticulocyte count (%) of 0.08%. Serum iron was 32.1 μmol/L; transferrin saturation was 90.7%; ferritin was 534.8 μg/L; folic acid was >54.48 nmol/L; and vitamin B_{12} was 436 pmol/L, indicating that he had no obvious iron, folic acid, or vitamin B12 deficiency. To explore the cause of anemia, bone marrow puncture was performed. The result revealed that erythroid hematopoiesis was reduced in the bone marrow and then we speculated pure red cell aplastic disorder was a likely cause of anemia. However, the erythropoietin (EPO) antibodies was detected as negative.

The patient was then diagnosed EPO-induced pure red cell aplastic anemia (PRCA) and treated with roxadustat at a dosage of 120 mg three times per week instead of EPO combined with iron supplementation. Immunosuppressive therapy with 50 mg cyclosporine twice a day was started on January 28, 2021. Later, as anemia was still present, the dosage of cyclosporine was increased to 100 mg twice a day on March 10, 2021, and 40 mg of testosterone undecanoate was administered thrice a day. From April 2021 to May 2022, the hemoglobin concentration increased gradually; testosterone undecanoate was stopped; cyclosporine was reduced to 25 mg twice a day; Wuzhi capsules were used to increase the blood concentration of cyclosporine, and the roxadustat dosage was reduced to 100 mg three times per week. When the hemoglobin level increased to 105 g/L on June 21, 2022 and 108 g/L on July 11, 2022, the Wuzhi capsules were stopped. Next, the cyclosporine dosage was reduced to 25 mg once a day when the hemoglobin level reached 114 g/L on September 5, 2022. During the follow-up from October 2022 to March 2023, the patient's hemoglobin levels were maintained at 100–115 g/L. On April 26, 2023, the hemoglobin level decreased to 77 g/L, and the trough value of the

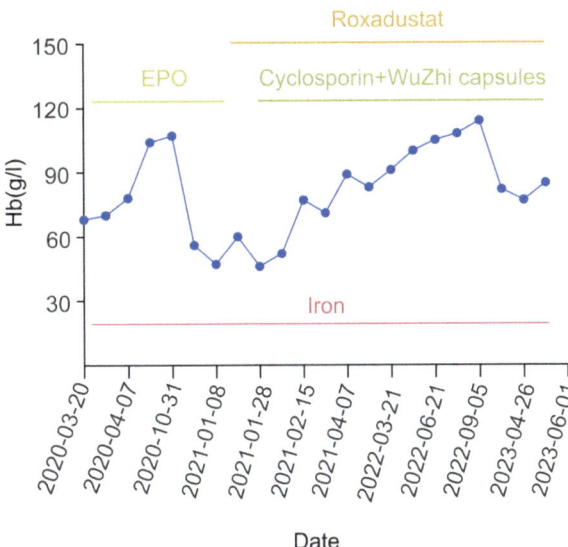

Fig. 17.1 Changes in hemoglobin levels

cyclosporine plasma concentration was less than 25 pg/ml; therefore, Wuzhi capsules were used again. On May 12, 2023, the trough value of the plasma concentration of cyclosporine reached 199.7 pg/ml, while the hemoglobin concentration increased to 85 g/L. These findings indicate that the use of cyclosporine combined with Wuzhi capsules has significant efficacy for the treatment of EPO-induced PRCA (Fig. 17.1).

17.2 Discussion

This elderly male patient who underwent regular peritoneal dialysis presented with moderate to severe anemia, and his hemoglobin gradually increased to normal levels after receiving a high dose of EPO. However, 10 months later, severe anemia occurred again. On the basis of anemia recurrence and bone marrow aspiration results, the patient was diagnosed with EPO-induced PRCA. Then, his medication regimen was switched from EPO to roxadustat, with immunotherapy co-administration to treat anemia; later, his hemoglobin returned to normal levels.

Erythropoiesis-stimulating agents (ESAs) have been the mainstay of renal anemia treatment. However, clinical treatment is still difficult, as some patients are hyporesponsive. The most common causes of hyporesponsiveness are iron deficiency, infection or inflammation, inadequate dialysis, severe hyperparathyroidism, malignancy, and bone marrow disease, among others [1]. When screening for potential causes of ESA hyporesponsiveness, clinicians also need to focus on the possibility of EPO-related PRCA [2, 3]. For this patient, we first screened for several common causes and found no relevant risk factors. Then, we performed a bone marrow examination, and the report showed that erythroid hematopoiesis was reduced and that a pure red cell aplastic disorder was likely. Moreover, the EPO antibody test result was negative, and we mainly considered this to be a false-negative result caused by low antibody affinity or low reagent sensitivity [4]. On the basis of severe anemia reappearance 10 months after ESA treatment, as well as reticulocytopenia, no iron deficiency, and bone marrow aspiration results, we diagnosed the patient with EPO-induced PRCA and administered immunotherapy. His hemoglobin level began to recover after 2 months of treatment and reached 105 g/L after 5 months, which supported the diagnosis.

PRCA is a disease caused by erythroid hematopoietic failure that manifests only as anemia, such as decreased hemoglobin levels, reticulocytopenia, and extremely reduced or absent of erythroid precursor cells in the bone marrow. PRCA has a low morbidity and can be divided into congenital or acquired PRCA, and acquired PRCA is mostly related to tumors (thymomas), connective tissue diseases, viral infections, pregnancy, drugs, and EPO [5].

EPO-induced PRCA often occurs 3–4 weeks after EPO administration, with an average time of onset of 6–18 months after EPO treatment [3]. The patient was diagnosed at 10 months after treatment. Mechanistically, the drug induces the body to produce neutralizing antibodies to the EPO molecule [6]. According to approximately 200 reported cases of EPO-induced PRCA, almost all of them were chronic kidney disease patients who received subcutaneous administration of EPO, possibly due to the following reasons: (1) the risk of immunogenicity caused by the subcutaneous route of EPO administration; (2) the manufacturer of EPO replacing human blood albumin with polysorbate 80 in the formulation, which reduced the stability of the drug; (3) changes in the spatial structure of EPO due to storage conditions; (4) contamination from a small amount of silica gel, which is used to lubricate the prefilled syringe; and (5) the rubber stopper in the syringe possibly releasing some chemicals that act as immune adjuvants in the occurrence of disease [6–8].

At present, clinical experience in the treatment of EPO-induced PRCA remains to be limited, but it mainly includes the following:

1. Discontinuation of recombinant ESAs: It is recommended to discontinue all recombinant ESAs for patients with PRCA and to not switch to other ESAs.
2. Initial immunosuppressive therapy: As spontaneous remission rarely occurs after stopping recombinant ESAs, immunosuppressive therapy is often needed:
   (a) Initial treatment with prednisone [1 mg/(kg·d)] combined with oral cyclophosphamide (50–100 mg/d), which can be used for up to 3–4 months.
   (b) Another available alternative to first-line therapy is cyclosporine 200 mg/day (or 100 mg twice a day).
   (c) Tacrolimus can also be considered as a replacement to cyclosporine.
   (d) Intravenous infusion of immune globulin or rituximab, which is costly, potentially toxic, and has poor efficacy, so it may be limited to patients who do not respond to other treatments.
3. Kidney transplantation: The most effective treatment is kidney transplantation, which should be considered for patients for whom immunosuppressive therapy is ineffective and who are suitable candidates.

4. Follow-up anemia treatment: Hypoxia-inducible factor prolyl hydroxylase inhibitors (HIF-PHIs) can replace ESAs for the treatment of subsequent anemia in patients with EPO-induced PRCA [9–13].

Here, we report the case of a patient with EPO-induced PRCA, which is extremely rare. When progressive anemia occurs during the use of EPO, EPO-induced PRCA should be considered. We used roxadustat to replace ESA for anemia treatment, along with cyclosporine and Wuzhi capsules, which effectively and safely corrected anemia. This case provides a unique experience for treating patients with EPO-induced PRCA [13, 14].

References

1. Weir MR. Managing anemia across the stages of kidney disease in those hyporesponsive to erythropoiesis-stimulating agents. Am J Nephrol. 2021;52(6):450–66.
2. Casadevall N, Cournoyer D, Marsh J, et al. Recommendations on haematological criteria for the diagnosis of epoetin-induced pure red cell aplasia. Eur J Haematol. 2004;73(6):389–96.
3. Rossert J, Casadevall N, Eckardt KU. Anti-erythropoietin antibodies and pure red cell aplasia. J Am Soc Nephrol. 2004;15(2):398–406.
4. Thorpe R, Swanson SJ. Assays for detecting and diagnosing antibody-mediated pure red cell aplasia (PRCA): an assessment of available procedures. Nephrol Dial Transplant. 2005;20(Suppl 4):iv16–22.
5. Means RT. Pure red cell aplasia. Blood. 2016;128(21):2504–9.
6. Bunn HF. Drug-induced autoimmune red-cell aplasia. N Engl J Med. 2002;346(7):522–3.
7. Locatelli F, Del Vecchio L, Pozzoni P. Pure red-cell aplasia "epidemic"—mystery completely revealed? Perit Dial Int. 2007;27(Suppl 2):S303–7.
8. Padhi S, Panda SK. Acquired pure red cell aplasia and recombinant erythropoietin. Indian J Nephrol. 2021;31(4):331–5.
9. Cai KD, Zhu BX, Lin HX, Luo Q. Successful application of roxadustat in the treatment of patients with anti-erythropoietin antibody-mediated renal anaemia: a case report and literature review. J Int Med Res. 2021;49(4):3000605211005984.
10. Hashimoto K, Harada M, Kamijo Y. Pure red cell aplasia induced by anti-erythropoietin antibodies, well-controlled with tacrolimus. Int J Hematol. 2016;104(4):502–5.
11. Rossert J, Macdougall I, Casadevall N. Antibody-mediated pure red cell aplasia (PRCA) treatment and re-treatment: multiple options. Nephrol Dial Transplant. 2005;20(Suppl 4):iv23–6.
12. Verhelst D, Rossert J, Casadevall N, Krüger A, Eckardt KU, Macdougall IC. Treatment of erythropoietin-induced pure red cell aplasia: a retrospective study. Lancet. 2004;363(9423):1768–71.
13. Wu Y, Cai X, Ni J, Lin X. Resolution of epoetin-induced pure red cell aplasia, successful re-challenge with roxadustat. Int J Lab Hematol. 2020;42(6):e291–3.
14. Li S, Chen X, Hu P, et al. Roxadustat improves erythropoietin antibody-mediated pure red cell aplasia in a patient with hemodialysis. Blood Purif. 2022;51(2):189–92.

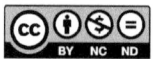

Roxadustat for the Treatment of Erythropoietin-Hyporesponsive Anemia in a Hemodialysis Patient: A Case Report

18

Huizi Zhu, Xiaowei Yang, and Rong Wang

18.1 Case Presentation

A 72-year-old man developed hyperglycemia approximately 20 years prior to admission. He did not accept any hypoglycemic drugs, and his blood glucose control status was unknown. A higher serum creatinine (Scr) level of 161 µmol/L was found 7 years prior to presentation, with thrombocytopenia, occasional gingival bleeding, and intermittent treatment with oral caffeic acid tablets. Approximately 18 months prior to admission, his Scr level increased to 569 µmol/L, and his hemoglobin (Hb) level decreased to 63 g/L. Maintenance hemodialysis (thrice weekly) and recombinant human erythropoietin (rhuEPO, 4000 U, three times weekly) were given. Approximately 2 months prior to admission, the patient suffered from recurrent fatigue, and a hematological examination revealed an Hb level of 45 g/L. After a 4-U red blood cell transfusion, the Hb level increased to 69 g/L. The rhuEPO dosage was adjusted to 8000 U three times weekly, and rhuEPO was combined with sucrose iron (0.1 g, intravenous drip, two times weekly). The patient suffered from decreased blood pressure and dizziness during hemodialysis 2 weeks prior, and his blood pressure gradually increased after the end of hemodialysis. The patient was subsequently admitted to the 960th Hospital of PLA. Hematological examination revealed an Hb level of 48 g/L and a PLT count of 102×10^9/L. Multiple fecal occult blood test showed positive, and bone marrow biopsy revealed no obvious abnormalities. After an 8-U red blood cell transfusion, his Hb level increased to 63 g/L. Four days later, the Hb level decreased to 45 g/L again. To further treat anemia, he was admitted to our department on January 13, 2020.

He had more than 9-year history of hypertension and regularly took "Adalat and irbesartan." The blood pressure reached 270/100 mmHg. He also had an 8-year history of coronary heart disease and two stents implanted. No anticoagulant or

H. Zhu · X. Yang · R. Wang (✉)
Shandong Provincial Hospital Affiliated to Shandong First Medical University,
Jinan, Shandong, China

© The Author(s) 2025
B.-C. Liu (ed.), *Treatment of Refractory Renal Anemia*,
https://doi.org/10.1007/978-981-97-7636-8_18

109

antiplatelet drugs were taken. He had more than 7-year history of thrombocytopenia, occasional gingival bleeding, and intermittent use of "caffeic acid tablets." He
underwent blood transfusions because of severe anemia. He also had more than
20-year history of smoking and 20-year history of drinking, but had already stopped
drinking for 1 year. No other special information was noted in his personal or family
history. His blood pressure was 132/62 mmHg, and his weight was 62 kg. Physical
examination revealed a very pale face. The heart rhythm is regular, and no pathological murmurs are heard in the auscultation areas of the valves. The breathing
sounds in both lungs are clear, with no dry or moist rales heard. There is no edema
throughout the body.

After admission, hematological examination revealed an Hb level of 48 g/L, a
PLT count of 53×10^9/L, a reticulocyte ratio of 7.7%, a mean erythrocyte hemoglobin concentration (MCHC) of 323 g/L, and normal blood cell morphology. The
serum ferritin concentration was 1170 μg/L; transferrin saturation was 57%; the
level of erythropoietin was 84 mIU/mL, and the concentration levels of folic acid
and VitB$_{12}$ were higher than the normal ranges. Fecal occult blood test results were
−/+. The level of albumin was 29.8 g/L; the Scr level was 890 μmol/L, and the parathyroid hormone (PTH) level was 34.27 ng/L. Tumor marker levels were within
normal ranges. The results of an antiglobulin test (Coombs test), acid hemolysis test
(Ham's test), and sucrose hemolysis test were all negative. Abdominal ultrasonography revealed bilateral atrophic kidneys and a spleen thickness of 4.5 cm. Cardiac
ultrasound and chest computed tomography (CT) showed no obvious
abnormalities.

For treatment, blood transfusion, rhuEPO (10,000 U, three times weekly), and
adequate dialysis three times weekly were given. Hb increased to 72 g/L on January
17 and then decreased again to 43 g/L on January 22 (Fig. 18.1 shows the Hb
changes in the patient during rhuEPO treatment). Red blood cells (3.5 U) were
infused on January 23. Considering the poor response to rhuEPO, we recommended

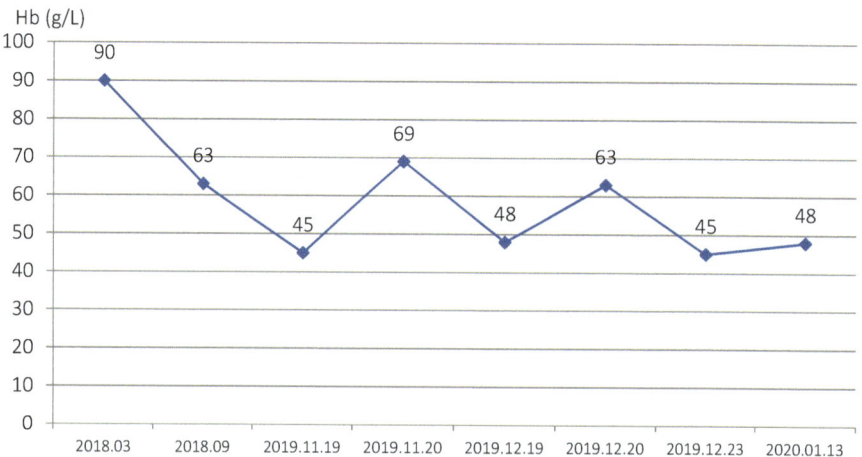

Fig. 18.1 Hb changes in the patient before treatment with rhuEPO

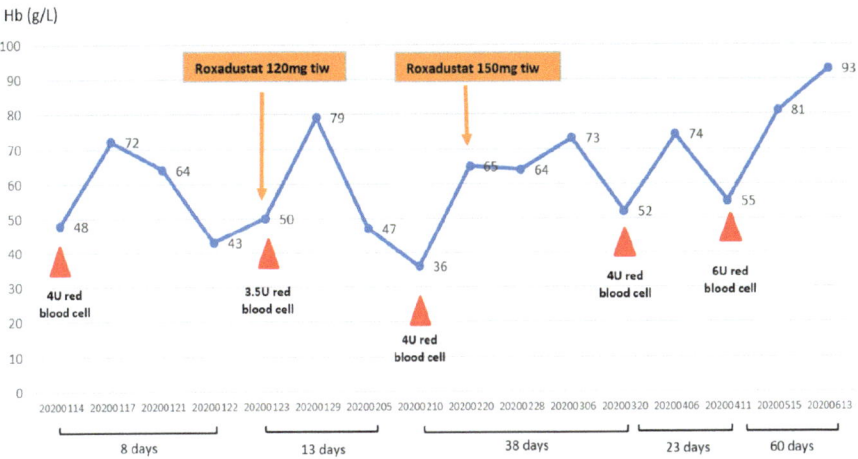

Fig. 18.2 Hb changes after treatment with roxadustat

the administration of roxadustat (120 mg, three times weekly) orally to treat his anemia. Although the interval between blood transfusions was prolonged after roxadustat treatment, his Hb level decreased to 47 g/L again on February 5. After red blood cell infusion, the dosage of roxadustat was adjusted to 150 mg (three times weekly), and his Hb level increased to 73 g/L after 2 weeks. Afterward, his Hb level fluctuated between ~50 and 75 g/L, during which time the patient was given two red blood cell transfusions. The Hb concentration began to increase continuously beginning in May and reached 93 g/L on June 13, 2020 (Fig. 18.2 shows the changes in Hb after roxadustat treatment).

18.2   Discussion

In this case, roxadustat was used for the treatment of erythropoiesis-stimulating agent (ESA) hyporesponsiveness-related anemia in a maintenance hemodialysis patient. Despite treatment with 24,000 IU rhuEPO weekly (patient's weight was 62 kg), the patient still required repeated blood transfusion, and his Hb decreased rapidly in a short time. This patient had anemia with thrombocytopenia, but no obvious abnormality was found with two bone marrow biopsies; the proportion of reticulocytes was high, and no evidence of hematological diseases as a cause of anemia was found. There was no iron deficiency or iron utilization disorder in this patient according to the results of ferritin and transferrin saturation. His C-reactive protein (CRP) level was normal, and there was no obvious infection; therefore, ESA hyporesponsiveness caused by infection could be excluded. Moreover, there was no evidence of secondary hyperparathyroidism or hemolytic anemia in this patient. Many fecal occult blood tests were positive; the patient did not undergo gastrointestinal endoscopy due to weakness; also, we are not certain if this patient's refractory anemia is caused by gastrointestinal blood loss, although there was no obvious black stool or hematochezia. This patient has thrombocytopenia, but the platelet count has been stable around $50 \times 10^9/L$, and, on one occasion, when there was a rapid decrease in hemoglobin, the platelet count was $90 \times 10^9/L$. Therefore, the rapid decrease in hemoglobin in this patient does not seem to be caused by bleeding due to low platelet levels. During the process of dialysis, there was no coagulation of the dialyzer and no bleeding from the digestive tract. This case was rare in that the patient still needed frequent blood transfusions after rhuEPO treatment. Despite the cause of the refractory anemia being unclear, it was surprising that following treatment with roxadustat, there was a notable reduction in the frequency of blood transfusions and a decrease in the dosage of iron required, while the hemoglobin levels experienced a significant increase.

huEPO combined with iron has been the main treatment for patients with renal anemia. The China Clinical Practice Guide for Diagnosis and Treatment of Renal Anemia of 2021 defined ESA hyporesponsiveness initial treatment as the inability to achieve or maintain target Hb levels through an appropriate ESA dose based on body weight for 1 month. Acquired ESA hyporesponsiveness is defined as an increase in the ESA dose by two times and an increase in the dose of more than 50% of the stable dose to maintain target Hb levels [1]. It was still difficult to achieve or maintain target Hb levels in this patient, and frequent blood transfusions were needed despite the use of higher than usual doses of ESAs. ESA hyporesponsiveness was considered in this patient.

ESA hyporesponsiveness is common in patients with oxidative stress, inflammatory state, iron deficiency, hematological diseases, certain drug use (such as angiotensin-converting enzyme inhibitors [ACEIs] and angiotensin II receptor blockers [ARBs]), aluminum poisoning, secondary hyperparathyroidism, and so on [2]. This patient had no obvious inflammatory state, no absolute or relative iron deficiency, and no secondary hyperparathyroidism or other common causes of ESA hyporesponsiveness. After switching the medication regimen to roxadustat, the intervals between blood transfusions gradually lengthened, and a stable Hb level was achieved.

At the initial stage of roxadustat treatment, the Hb level was monitored every 2 weeks until it stabilized, after which it was monitored every 4 weeks. The dose of roxadustat should be adjusted according to the Hb level to maintain the Hb level at $100 \sim 120$ g/L and minimize the need for blood transfusion. Blood pressure, iron metabolism, and Hb levels were monitored at the beginning of treatment. The patient did not achieve a target Hb level at the recommended roxadustat dosage (120 mg, three times weekly). To minimize the need for blood transfusion, we adjusted the roxadustat dosage to 150 mg three times weekly.

In patients with ESA hyporesponsiveness-related anemia, it is difficult to achieve or maintain target Hb levels, and these patients often have a poor prognosis because high-dose ESAs increase the risk of adverse cardiovascular events [3, 4]. Fortunately, roxadustat was effective in correcting anemia in dialysis patients [5, 6]. Roxadustat can directly regulate the endogenous EPO gene expression to significantly increase the level of Hb in patients with renal anemia; its efficacy is unaffected by iron metabolism and the inflammatory state, and it treats renal anemia. The efficacy of roxadustat in this patient suggested that it would be an alternative therapy for those with ESA hyporesponsiveness in renal anemia. Clearly, as the mechanistically new type of drug for renal anemia, it is worthwhile to further understand its unique role in the treatment of renal anemia.

References

1. Chinese Nephrologist Association Renal Anemia Guideline Working Group. The clinical practice guidelines for diagnosis and treatment of renal anemia in China. Natl Med J China. 2021;101(20):1463–502.
2. Bamgbola OF. Pattern of resistance to erythropoietin-stimulating agents in chronic kidney disease. Kidney Int. 2011;80(5):464–74.
3. Solomon SD, Uno H, Lewis EF, et al. Erythropoietic response and outcomes in kidney disease and type 2 diabetes. N Engl J Med. 2010;363(12):1146–55.
4. Szczech LA, Barnhart HX, Inrig JK, et al. Secondary analysis of the CHOIR trial epoetin-alpha dose and achieved hemoglobin outcomes. Kidney Int. 2008;74(6):791–8.
5. Chen N, Hao C, Liu BC, et al. Roxadustat treatment for anemia in patients undergoing long-term dialysis. N Engl J Med. 2019;381(11):1011–22.
6. Chen N, Hao C, Peng X, et al. Roxadustat for anemia in patients with kidney disease not receiving dialysis. N Engl J Med. 2019;381(11):1001–10.

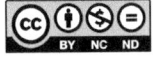

Part IV

CKD Anemia Combined with Other Complex Diseases

End-stage kidney disease (ESKD) is a clinically complex syndrome. Owing to the multiple functions of kidney in nature and the very complicated primary causes of kidney disease, patients with ESKD are commonly faced with tough situations, including refractory renal anemia. In addition, patients also have other complicated systemic diseases, which sometimes are very challenging to renal physicians. It is well recognized that poor correction of hemoglobin not only impacts the patient's quality of life, but more importantly, it can lead to high morbidity and mortality. It is therefore always important for physicians to find a way to overcome the difficulties that guidelines or clinical trials may not fully address. For the clinical, practice is sometimes ahead of theory. In this part, we provide several interesting clinical cases, with the aim of stimulating clinical decision-making for the management of patients with more complex severe renal anemia.

Treatment of Severe Anemia in a Hemodialysis Patient with Bone Marrow Hypoplasia

Zuo-Lin Li and Bi-Cheng Liu

19.1 Case Presentation

A 53-year-old woman was in her usual health until approximately 6 years before admission, when a diagnosis of "diabetic nephropathy" was made because of the edema in her lower extremities accompanied by foam in her urine. Five months prior to admission, a diagnosis of "chronic kidney disease (CKD) stage 5 and diabetic nephropathy (stage 5)" was made, with worsening symptoms and significantly elevated serum creatinine levels. She was initially treated with hemodialysis three times per week after an arteriovenous fistula was established. In addition, she received intravenous recombinant human erythropoietin (r-HuEPO) at a dosage of 3000 U three times per week for her anemia (with hemoglobin concentrations ranging from 6.0 to 7.0 g/dL). Three months prior to admission, she complained of significant dizziness and fatigue, having a hemoglobin concentration of 5.9 g/dL; therefore, blood transfusion and iron supplementation were given to correct anemia. Moreover, the dose of r-HuEPO was adjusted to 16,000 U/week. However, r-HuEPO efficacy against anemia remained poor. Two months prior to admission, the patient's medication was switched to roxadustat at a dosage of 100 mg three times per week and then to roxadustat at a dosage of 120 mg three times per week after 1 month due to poor efficacy results (with hemoglobin concentrations ranging from 5.5 to 6.0 g/dL).

Z.-L. Li
Institute of Nephrology, Zhong Da Hospital, Southeast University School of Medicine, Nanjing, China

B.-C. Liu (✉)
Institute of Nephrology, Zhongda Hospital, Southeast University, Nanjing, China

© The Author(s) 2025   117
B.-C. Liu (ed.), *Treatment of Refractory Renal Anemia*,
https://doi.org/10.1007/978-981-97-7636-8_19

The patient had a 20-year history of diabetes, which was treated with subcutaneous administration of recombinant insulin. She also had a 10-year history of hypertension, for which she regularly took antihypertensive drugs (nifedipine controlled-release tablets). She also had a cholecystectomy 20 years prior to admission. No other special information was noted regarding her personal or family history. Her blood pressure was 171/86 mmHg, and her body weight was 59 kg. Physical examination revealed a very pale face, an enlarged cardiac boundary, and mild pitting edema in both lower extremities.

Laboratory examinations revealed the following: white blood cell (WBC) count, 5.4×10^9/L; red blood cell (RBC) count, 2.09×10^{12}/L; hemoglobin, 61 g/L; platelet count, 79×10^9/L; reticulocyte count, 9.93×10^{10}/L; C-reactive protein, 8.58 mg/L; total serum protein, 60.5 g/L; albumin, 40.4 g/L; blood urea nitrogen, 32.8 mmol/L; creatinine, 852 μmol/L (reference range, 57–111 μmol/L); serum calcium, 2.25 mmol/L; phosphorus, 1.66 mmol/L; and uric acid, 457 μmol/L. Serological test results for tumor markers, autoantibodies (including anti-nuclear, anti-double-stranded DNA, anti-glomerular basement membrane, and anti-neutrophil cytoplasmic antibodies), and viral infections (hepatitis B and C or HIV infections) were all negative. Moreover, there was no evidence of hematological disease (serum protein electrophoresis and immunofixation electrophoresis) or hemolytic disease (Coombs test, CD55, and CD59 expression). Ultrasonography of the abdomen revealed nonspecific mild splenomegaly (12.73 cm × 4.0 cm). In addition, her nutritional status was good, and her parathyroid hormone level was controlled within the appropriate range for hemodialysis patients (intact parathyroid hormone: 171 ~ 371 pg/mL).

In addition, biomarkers of iron status, including stored iron and functional iron, were measured. Interestingly, she had no obvious iron deficiency (iron, 10.3 μmol/L; transferrin saturation, 12.50%; total iron-binding capacity, 82.4 μmol/L; and ferritin 271.05 μg/L). To determine the cause of anemia, bone marrow puncture was performed. Interestingly, bone marrow hypoplasia was found with anisocytosis, as well as a granulocyte percentage of 71%. No other distinguishing abnormalities were observed.

Treatment involved intensive hemodialysis with strict control of blood glucose and blood pressure. Given the patient's past medical history and clinical use of roxadustat, we prescribed a dose of roxadustat of 150 mg three times per week, and the hemoglobin level was noted to increase gradually to 9.8 g/dL after 1 month. During the 3-month follow-up, the patient's hemoglobin levels were maintained at approximately 10 g/dL with the same dosage of roxadustat (Fig. 19.1).

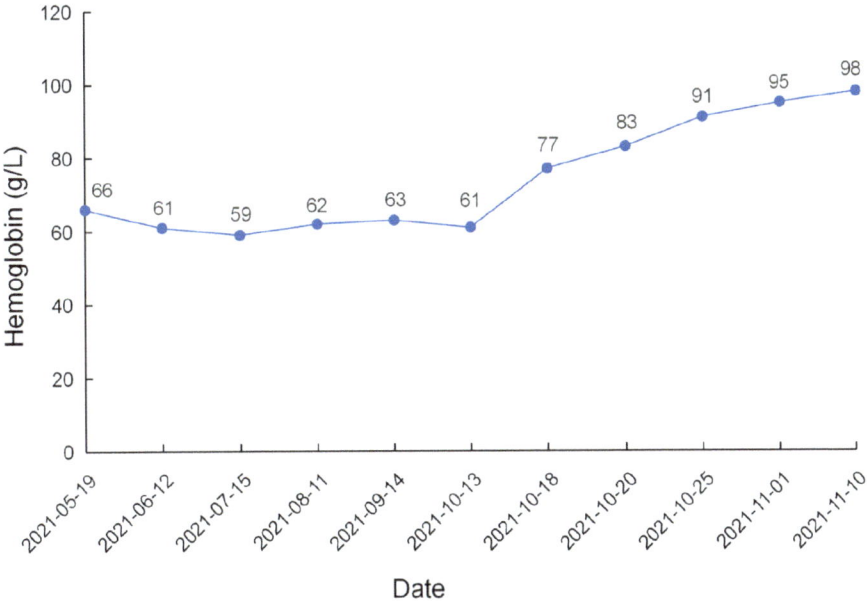

Fig. 19.1 Changes in hemoglobin levels

19.2 Discussion

This case involves a middle-aged female patient on regular hemodialysis who presented with moderate to severe anemia and a history of type 2 diabetes and hypertension. Before hospitalization, a high dose of EPO supplement was given, but the patient seemed unresponsive. Then, the patient's medication was switched from EPO to roxadustat, and the dosage of roxadustat was adjusted according to the instructions. Unfortunately, the patient was still hyporesponsive in the initial stage, and the hemoglobin level remained at 5.5 ~ 6.0 g/dL. Therefore, this patient was characterized as having erythropoiesis-stimulating agent (ESA) hyporesponsiveness.

ESAs have been the mainstay of renal anemia treatment; however, an unmet clinical need remains, owing to the hyporesponsive population. Although disease severity and comorbidities may, in part, contribute to ESA hyporesponsiveness, the most common causes of ESA hyporesponsiveness include iron deficiency, inflammation, secondary hyperparathyroidism, and inadequate dialysis [1]. Therefore, we screened the patient for factors that may contribute to ESA hyporesponsiveness. Notably, bone marrow puncture revealed bone marrow hypoplasia with anisocytosis.

Despite multiple factors associated with ESA hyporesponsiveness in patients with CKD, it is important to keep in mind that EPO-associated pure red cell aplasia may be one of the potential causes of severe anemia. For this patient, although we did not detect anti-EPO antibodies, the morphological changes in the bone marrow did not support this hypothesis. Here, due to the poor therapeutic effect of ESA supplementation, the patient's medication was switched to roxadustat, which has a novel mechanism of action in the treatment of anemia. Unfortunately, she also showed poor response to the conventional recommended dose of roxadustat. To date, clinicians have prescribed roxadustat mainly according to the experiences gained in phase II and III clinical studies. Based on the results of clinical trials, the therapeutic effect of roxadustat was dose dependent [2, 3]. Therefore, the roxadustat dosage was titrated gradually to 150 mg three times per week. Fortunately, the patient's hemoglobin level increased gradually and has remained within a relatively reasonable range during follow-up.

Sometimes, it is difficult to make a definitive diagnosis of the cause of anemia, which is likely to be multifactorial [4, 5]. Although hematological diseases (aplastic anemia, myelodysplastic syndromes, or other hematological diseases) could not be excluded as a cause of anemia in this patient, bone marrow suppression due to uremic toxins is perhaps the most common cause of unexplained anemia. Notably, the use of high-dose ESAs increases the risk of cardiovascular events and death; therefore, finding new strategies for treating anemia in patients with ESA hyporesponsiveness is an unmet need.

As a new-generation drug for the treatment of renal anemia with a novel mechanism, roxadustat is an orally bioavailable hypoxia-inducible factor prolyl hydroxylase inhibitor that mimics the natural response to hypoxia [6, 7]. Interestingly, roxadustat has become an attractive alternative treatment, especially for patients with ESA hyporesponsiveness. Mechanistically, roxadustat promotes not only endogenous EPO production and iron absorption, transport, and utilization but also the expression of the EPO receptor on erythroid progenitor cells [8], which may explain the beneficial effect of roxadustat observed in this rare case of anemia.

Roxadustat has been in clinical use for 4 years; thus, extensive clinical experience has been achieved [9]. According to clinical practice, roxadustat may correct anemia independent of bone marrow status. However, although clinical trials aiming to explore the efficacy and safety of roxadustat for treating anemia in patients with myelodysplastic syndrome have been completed [10], the therapeutic efficacy of roxadustat for CKD patients with bone marrow hypoplasia remains to be poorly understood.

Here, we report the case of an anemic patient with bone marrow hypoplasia who exhibited a poor response to high-dose ESAs. Although the dosage of roxadustat used was greater than the conventional recommended dosage, roxadustat corrected anemia effectively and safely. Therefore, this case provides a unique experience for the use of this new class of drug to treat patients with ESA hyporesponsiveness.

References

1. Wu HHL, Chinnadurai R. Erythropoietin-stimulating agent hyporesponsiveness in patients living with chronic kidney disease. Kidney Dis (Basel). 2022;8(2):103–14.
2. Provenzano R, Besarab A, Sun CH, et al. Oral hypoxia-inducible factor prolyl hydroxylase inhibitor roxadustat (FG-4592) for the treatment of anemia in patients with CKD. Clin J Am Soc Nephrol. 2016;11(6):982–91.
3. Provenzano R, Besarab A, Wright S, et al. Roxadustat (FG-4592) versus epoetin alfa for anemia in patients receiving maintenance hemodialysis: a phase 2, randomized, 6- to 19-week, open-label, active-comparator, dose-ranging, safety and exploratory efficacy study. Am J Kidney Dis. 2016;67(6):912–24.
4. Babitt JL, Lin HY. Mechanisms of anemia in CKD. J Am Soc Nephrol. 2012;23(10):1631–4.
5. Babitt JL, Lin HY. Molecular mechanisms of hepcidin regulation: implications for the anemia of CKD. Am J Kidney Dis. 2010;55(4):726–41.
6. Schödel J, Ratcliffe PJ. Mechanisms of hypoxia signalling: new implications for nephrology. Nat Rev Nephrol. 2019;15(10):641–59.
7. Anker MS, Butler J, Anker SD. Roxadustat for anemia in patients with chronic kidney disease. N Engl J Med. 2020;383(1):e3.
8. Li ZL, Tu Y, Liu BC. Treatment of renal anemia with roxadustat: advantages and achievement. Kidney Dis (Basel). 2020;6(2):65–73.
9. Nephrology Committee of Chinese Research Hospital Association. Chinese expert consensus on the treatment of renal anemia with Roxadustat. Natl Med J China. 2022;102(24):1802–10.
10. Henry DH, Glaspy J, Harrup R, et al. Roxadustat for the treatment of anemia in patients with lower-risk myelodysplastic syndrome: open-label, dose-selection, lead-in stage of a phase 3 study. Am J Hematol. 2022;97(2):174–84.

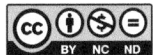

Treatment of Severe Renal Anemia in a Hemodialysis Patient with Decompensation of Liver Cirrhosis and Irregular Positive Erythrocyte Antibody

20

Feng-Mei Wang, Yan-Tu, and Bin Wang

20.1 Case Presentation

A 56-year-old woman was admitted to our hospital due to intermittent and worsening tarry stools for 20 days. The woman was a hemodialysis patient. She was diagnosed with chronic nephritis and foam in her urine 30 and 25 years prior to admission, respectively. She had to terminate her pregnancy at 6 months because of progressive deterioration of renal function to end-stage renal disease (ESRD), after which she started maintenance hemodialysis three times per week. Twenty-one years prior to admission, she briefly went off hemodialysis because she received a kidney transplant. Unfortunately, the transplanted kidney stopped functioning only 2 years later, and she then resumed regular hemodialysis. Four months after she resumed hemodialysis, she was diagnosed with "massive gastrointestinal bleeding" because of the decompensation of liver cirrhosis and urgently underwent transjugular intrahepatic portosystemic shunt (TIPS) surgery in the same year. The surgery went smoothly; her overall condition improved, and she no longer had hematemesis or tarry stools, but her moderate anemia persisted. Approximately 20 days prior to admission, she experienced tarry stools again, which persisted and continued to worsen, as mentioned earlier. The patient had positive fecal occult blood test results, worsening anemia (hemoglobin, 55 g/L), and decreased blood pressure (80/45 mmHg). Before hospitalization, she received intravenous recombinant human erythropoietin (r-HuEPO) at a dosage of 3000 U three times per week and 150 mg of polysaccharide iron complex capsules orally once a day for treating anemia.

F.-M. Wang · Yan-Tu
Institute of Nephrology, Zhong Da Hospital, Southeast University School of Medicine, Nanjing, China

B. Wang (✉)
Institute of Nephrology, Zhongda Hospital, Southeast University, Nanjing, China

© The Author(s) 2025
B.-C. Liu (ed.), *Treatment of Refractory Renal Anemia*,
https://doi.org/10.1007/978-981-97-7636-8_20

The patient had a 30-year history of hypertension, with a maximum blood pressure of 220/110 mmHg. Three years prior to admission, due to secondary hyperparathyroidism, she underwent total parathyroidectomy. Her blood pressure gradually decreased, and antihypertensive drugs were discontinued, with her blood pressure fluctuating at 80–110/(60–90) mmHg. She also had a 10-year history of coronary heart disease and underwent left main artery and left anterior descending branch stent implantation. Furthermore, she had a history of hepatitis C 15 years prior to admission, and after 2 years of treatment, she became negative for hepatitis C virus RNA in the year prior to admission. No other special information was noted in her personal or family history. On admission, her blood pressure was 88/60 mmHg, and her body weight was 51 kg. Physical examination revealed a very pale face, an enlarged cardiac boundary, and a moderately enlarged spleen.

Laboratory examinations revealed the following: white blood cell (WBC) count, 6.31×10^9/L; red blood cell (RBC) count, 2.08×10^{12}/L; hemoglobin, 49 g/L; platelet count, 86×10^9/L; neutrophil percentage, 81.31%; total serum protein, 54.1 g/L; albumin, 28.9 g/L; creatinine, 388 μmol/L; prothrombin time (PT), 13.10 s; activated partial thromboplastin time (APTT), 27.50 s; international normalized ratio (INR), 1.22; plasma fibrinogen (FIB), 2.37 g/L; D-dimer, 1813 μg/L; high-sensitivity C-reactive protein, 79 mm/L; and Coombs test, (+). No obvious abnormalities were found in other laboratory examination indicators. Ultrasonography of the abdomen revealed nonspecific moderate splenomegaly (17.40 cm × 5.70 cm).

After a multidisciplinary team (MDT) considered the patient's critical and complex condition and many basic diseases, they suggested and implemented conventional and conservative medical management, including fasting and water deprivation, nutritional support, inhibition of gastric acid secretion, somatostatin hemostasis, continuous renal replacement therapy (CRRT), anti-infection treatment, and intravenous recombinant human erythropoietin (r-HuEPO) at a dosage of 3000 U three times per week. After treatment, the overall condition of the patient improved, but her symptoms of dizziness and palpitations did not improve within a short period. In addition, her hemoglobin level continued to decrease, with a minimum value of 43 g/L. In particular, the patient had type O blood and was positive for irregular red blood cell antibodies. Multiple blood matching attempts were unsuccessful, and blood transfusion was not possible.

In addition, starting from the sixth day after admission, roxadustat was given three times per week (100 mg) for treatment. One month later, a follow-up examination revealed a hemoglobin level of 62 g/L and fewer episodes of palpitations and dizziness, and the patient was discharged. During the follow-up period, the dosage of roxadustat was adjusted based on the patient's hemoglobin level as the Chinese roxadustat drug user manual. During the follow-up period, due to the recurrence of gastrointestinal bleeding, the patient's hemoglobin decreased to 63 g/L. After symptomatic treatment and oral administration of roxadustat, her hemoglobin levels gradually increased. During the follow-up period, multiple fecal occult blood tests were conducted, with positive and negative results. Changes in hemoglobin levels and other related indicators are shown in Table 20.1 and Fig. 20.1.

Table 20.1 Levels of hemoglobin, C-reactive protein, erythropoietin, and ferritin during treatment

	Hemoglobin	C-reactive protein	Erythropoietin	Ferritin
	(g/L)	(mm/L)	(mU/ml)	(µg/g)
Before medication	43	79.00	346.25	13.10
Medication for 1 week	61	–	–	–
Medication for 2 weeks	58	0.82	87.62	8.50
Medication for 4 weeks	73	–	–	–
Medication for 8 weeks	91	–	–	–
Medication for 12 weeks	91	12.50	13.31	122.90
Medication for 24 weeks	84	21.58	136.80	20.20
Medication for 12 months	79	44.10	45.90	65.60
Medication for 18 months	105	–	–	56.94

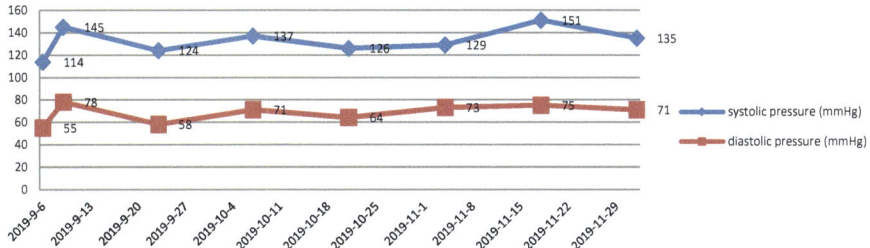

Fig. 20.1 Changes in blood pressure

20.2   Discussion

This middle-aged female, who is a long-term hemodialysis patient, presented with an acute exacerbation of chronic nephritis and uremia. The prominent clinical manifestation of this hospitalization was severe anemia. Moreover, she had a history of hepatitis C for many years, and antiviral treatment failed to prevent the progression of her condition to the decompensated stage of liver cirrhosis, complicated by hypersplenism, esophagofundus varicose veins, and recurrent gastrointestinal bleeding. She had received blood transfusions many times. Before hospitalization, a high dose of EPO supplement was given, but the patient seemed unresponsive. The difficulty in treating anemia in this patient was that acute blood loss caused by gastrointestinal bleeding and anemia caused by hypersplenism also occurred, in addition to renal anemia. However, due to the particularity of her own blood, allogeneic blood transfusion is impossible, and the classic "EPO+ chalybeate" program shows poor efficacy. If the anemia symptoms of the patient do not improve in the short term, the functions of multiple organs will be affected, which could be life-threatening.

Treatment with ESAs, chalybeate, and blood transfusions is the mainstay treatment for renal anemia, which significantly reduces the frequency and risk of blood transfusions in patients [1, 2]. At present, it is generally believed that the etiology of chronic kidney disease-related anemia is related not only to a deficiency of EPO and iron but also to an imbalance in iron homeostasis and excessive hepcidin, chronic inflammation, an impairment of renal oxygen perception mediated by hypoxia-inducible factor (HIF), hemolysis, blood loss, dialysis, the use of angiotensin-converting enzyme inhibitors (ACEIs), hyperparathyroidism, and so on [3].

Roxadustat, a representative hypoxia-inducible factor-prolyl hydroxylase inhibitor (HIF-PHI) that can comprehensively regulate the production of RBCs through multiple targets, correct anemia, and increase hemoglobin levels without being affected by microinflammation, is a new-generation drug for the treatment of renal anemia [4–6]. The condition of this patient was complex, involving an inflammatory state, iron deficiency, hypersplenism, acute blood loss, and limited blood transfusion. Although there is no reference case for roxadustat use in such patients worldwide, the analysis of indications for the use of roxadustat showed no obvious contraindications; therefore, the use of roxadustat in this patient with a complicated condition was recommended.

Routine blood examination was performed at week 1 and week 2 after treatment. The results showed that the hemoglobin level of the patient increased gradually, which confirmed that roxadustat indeed improved the patient's anemia. Subsequently, her hemoglobin level increased significantly and remained at 80 ~ 100 g/L without the need for blood transfusion despite adverse factors such as active bleeding and hypersplenism after discharge. During the treatment, she requested a roxadustat dose reduction due to economic reasons, resulting in a decrease in hemoglobin, which could still increase after roxadustat dose readjustment, indicating that the effect of roxadustat on hemoglobin levels is dose dependent. The iron reserve function of the patient was poor, and no intravenous iron supplementation was provided throughout the treatment but only intermittent oral chalybeate supplementation, suggesting that the ameliorating effect of roxadustat on anemia is relatively iron independent.

Here, we report a unique and complex case of a patient with uremia, anemia, a 25-year history of renal replacement therapy (including kidney transplantation), and comorbidities such as cirrhosis decompensation, hypersplenism, malnutrition, and gastrointestinal bleeding. In the treatment of anemia in such patients, it is important to correct these factors that may lead to EPO resistance [7]. More importantly, clinical transfusion was extremely difficult for her due to the presence of irregular RBC antibodies. Notably, anemia symptoms steadily resolved during the 1.5 years of observation after treatment with roxadustat.

Whether roxadustat also has a certain correcting effect on other factors related to EPO resistance (such as a microinflammatory state, erythrocyte antibody formation, and erythropoietin receptor) warrants further investigation, as does its ability to promote endogenous EPO release and increase iron metabolism [8–10].

Before the advent of roxadustat, the treatment of such patients was very difficult. Thus, this successful treatment provides a new reference for the treatment of similarly difficult renal anemia. In future clinical practice, it will be very important to observe not only the changes in hemoglobin levels but also changes in multiple iron metabolism indices and red blood cell antibody levels in a patient.

References

1. Li Y, Shi H, Wang WM, et al. Prevalence, awareness, and treatment of anemia in Chinese patients with nondialysis chronic kidney disease: first multicenter, cross-sectional study. Medicine (Baltimore). 2016;95(24):e3872.
2. Working group on renal anemia guidelines, branch of nephrology physicians, Chinese medical doctor association. Clinical practice guide for diagnosis and treatment of renal anemia in China. Chin Med J. 2021;101(20):1463–502.
3. Wish JB, Aronoff GR, Bacon BR, et al. Positive iron balance in chronic kidney disease: how much is too much and how to tell? Am J Nephrol. 2018;47(2):72–83.
4. Fu Y, Tu Y, Liu B. Research progress of hypoxic inducible factor - proline hydroxylase inhibitor in treatment of renal anemia. Chin J Nephrol. 2020;36(9):726–30.
5. Li ZL, Tu Y, Liu BC. Treatment of renal anemia with roxadustat: advantages and achievement. Kidney Dis (Basel). 2020;6(2):65–73.
6. Chen N, Hao C, Peng X, et al. Roxadustat for anemia in patients with kidney disease not receiving dialysis. N Engl J Med. 2019;381(11):1001–10.
7. Chen N, Hao C, Liu BC, et al. Roxadustat treatment for anemia in patients undergoing long-term dialysis. N Engl J Med. 2019;381(11):1011–22.
8. Tu Y, Zhang X. Clinical application of hypoxic-inducing factor prolyl hydroxylase inhibitor roxallistat. J Clin Ren Dis. 2020;20(7):594–7.
9. Pan M, Liu B. New progress of hypoxic inducible factor stabilizers in the treatment of renal anemia. Chin J Intern Med. 2017;56(3):225–8.
10. Del Balzo U, Signore PE, Walkinshaw G, et al. Nonclinical characterization of the hypoxia-inducible factor prolyl hydroxylase inhibitor roxadustat, a novel treatment of anemia of chronic kidney disease. J Pharmacol Exp Ther. 2020;374(2):342–53.

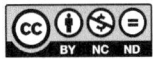

Treatment of Anemia in a Lupus Nephritis Patient with Renal Insufficiency, Infection, and Bone Marrow Hypoplasia

21

Min Wu, Ri-Ning Tang, and Bi-Cheng Liu

21.1 Case Presentation

A 39-year-old Chinese woman presented to the hospital with 1 month of facial erythema accompanied by bilateral lower limb swelling and foamy urine for 1 week. The results of her routine blood tests are as follows: white blood cell count (WBC), 3.71 × 10^9/L; hemoglobin (HGB), 72 g/L; platelet (PLT) count, 114 × 10^9/L; serum C3, 0.299 g/L; C4, 0.028 g/L; anti-double-stranded DNA (anti-dsDNA) titer, >800 IU/mL; serum creatine, 131 μmol/L; and urine protein, 3+. The patient was thereafter diagnosed with systemic lupus erythematosus (SLE) and lupus nephritis (LN). Methylprednisolone (MP) pulse therapy at a dose of 60 mg/day was administered for 1 week. However, the patient complained that the severity of lower limb swelling had worsened, and she experienced shortness of breath after activity began. The patient was thereafter transferred to the medical center of Southeast University Affiliated Zhongda Hospital.

After admission, a physical examination was performed. Facial erythema was primarily noted on both sides of the nose bridge and cheeks and was accompanied by hair loss and edema of the eyelids and lower limbs. Auscultation revealed crackles in the lower lung fields and dullness to percussion at the bases. The results of her routine blood tests were as follows: WBC count, 5.62 × 10^9/L; HGB, 56 g/L; PLT count, 54 × 10^9/L; ferritin, 353.65 μg/L; serum iron, 6.4 μmol/L; unsaturated iron, 24.1 μmol/L; transferrin saturation, 21%; total iron-binding capacity, 30.5 μmol/L; erythropoietin (EPO), 130.42 mIU/mL; anti-dsDNA titer, 770.25 IU/ml; anti-C1q antibody, >100 IU/mL; direct and indirect Coombs test, negative; serum C3,

M. Wu · R.-N. Tang · B.-C. Liu (✉)
Institute of Nephrology, Zhong Da Hospital, Southeast University School of Medicine, Nanjing, China

© The Author(s) 2025
B.-C. Liu (ed.), *Treatment of Refractory Renal Anemia*,
https://doi.org/10.1007/978-981-97-7636-8_21

0.254 g/L; C4, <0.0743 g/L; ADAMT13 activity, normal; antiphospholipid antibody, negative; erythrocyte sedimentation rate (ESR), 41 mm/h; TNF-α, 17.68 pg/mL; and albumin, 15.9 g/L. Renal dysfunction progressed, with 27.8 mmol/L urea and 350 μmol/L creatine. At the same time, the 24-h urine output decreased to 500–700 mL, and the 24-h urine total protein level was 7 g. A computed tomography (CT) scan revealed pleural, pericardial, and peritoneal effusion. Thus, continuous renal replacement (CRRT) and plasma exchange (PE) were initiated. The body weight of this patient was 70 kg. Moreover, MP intravenous therapy at a dose of 40 mg/day, oral hydroxychloroquine (0.1 g twice a day), mycophenolate mofetil (MMF, 0.25 g twice a day), and roxadustat (120 mg, three times per week) were given. After treatment, the patient's edema and dyspnea were attenuated. Subsequently, we performed renal biopsy. The results showed class IV + V LN, accompanied by acute tubular necrosis. Since the renal function and urine output of this patient had not recovered, hemodialysis treatment was continued at a frequency of three times per week.

Half a month later, the patient developed a fever, with a temperature between 37.8 and 38.5 °C, accompanied by severe cough without sputum. The results of her routine blood tests were as follows: WBC count, 1.99 × 10^9/L; HGB, 85 g/L; PLT count, 49 × 10^9/L; anti-dsDNA titer, 43.4 IU/mL; anti-C1q antibody, 29.2 IU/mL; serum C3, 0.609 g/L; C4, 0.145 g/L; albumin, 22.7 g/L; creatine, 308 μmol/L; and hemoculture, negative. Chest CT imaging revealed pleural effusion without obvious pulmonary infection. Bone marrow puncture was performed, and the findings indicated bone marrow hypoplasia. Thus, the fever was likely caused by an upper respiratory tract infection. The dose of MP was decreased to 24 mg/day. Moreover, γ-globulin infusions were given to improve immunity. Considering that MMF can induce bone marrow hypoplasia as a side effect, the administration of MMF was stopped. Subcutaneous injection of granulocyte colony-stimulating factor (G-CSF) and interleukin-11 was temporarily given to stimulate the production of WBCs and PLTs. During this process, hydroxychloroquine (0.1 g bid) and roxadustat (120 mg, three times per week) were continuously administered. After the body temperature decreased and remained within the normal range, a biologic agent telitacicept was added to control LN activity. Ten days later, routine blood tests revealed a WBC count of 6.31 × 10^9/L, a HGB level of 78 g/L, and a PLT count of 71 × 10^9/L.

Three months later, the urine output of this patient gradually increased to 1500–2000 mL/day. Renal function tests revealed that the serum creatine concentration had decreased to 139 μmol/L. Therefore, the hemodialysis treatment was suspended, and the tunneled cuffed catheter was removed. The results of her routine blood tests were as follows: WBC count, 4.43 × 10^9/L; HGB, 151 g/L; PLT count, 82 × 10^9/L; ferritin, 160 μg/L; serum iron, 15.4 μmol/L; unsaturated iron, 38 μmol/L; transferrin saturation, 28.8%; total iron-binding capacity, 53.4 μmol/L; EPO, 102.92 mIU/mL; anti-dsDNA titer, 15.82 IU/mL; anti-C1q antibody negativity, 0.908 g/L; C4, 0.0765 g/L; and albumin, 29.9 g/L. Then, the dosage of roxadustat was decreased to 50 mg three times per week. MP, hydroxychloroquine, and the biologic agent were continuously given to treat the LN.

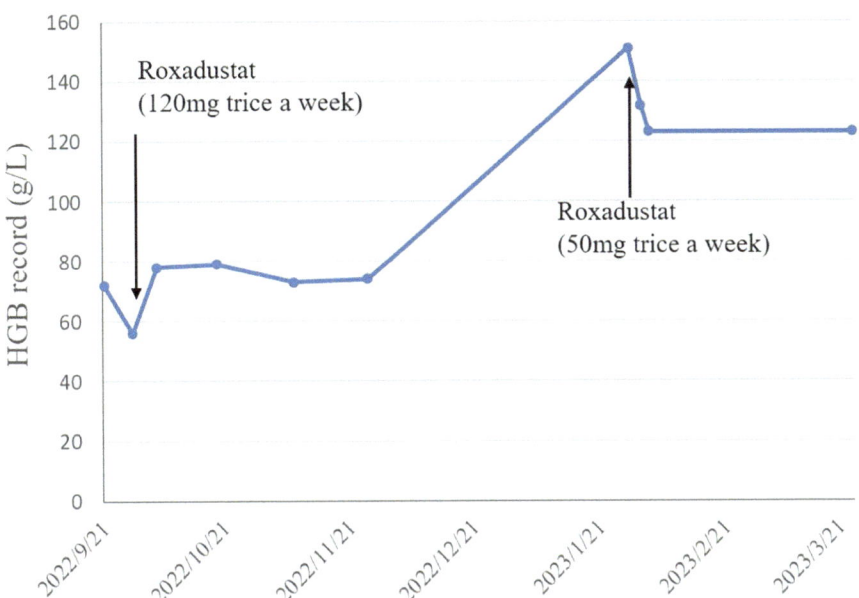

Fig. 21.1 Recorded HGB levels

Six months later, her routine blood tests revealed the following results: WBC count, $7.96 \times 10^9/L$; HGB, 123 g/L; PLT count, $97 \times 10^9/L$; ferritin, 278.08 µg/L; serum iron, 26.1 µmol/L; unsaturated iron, 31.7 µmol/L; transferrin saturation, 45.2%; total iron-binding capacity, 57.8 µmol/L; EPO, 86.19 mIU/mL; anti-dsDNA antibody titer, 0.941 g/L; serum C3, 0.0614 g/L; albumin, 33.2 g/L; creatine, 135 µmol/L; and 24 h-UTP, 0.943 g. MP was slowly tapered to a maintained dose of 8 mg/day. Roxadustat was maintained at a dosage of 50 mg three times per week (as shown in Fig. 21.1).

21.2   Discussion

Here, we described a 39-year-old female patient with SLE and LN suffering from complications of anemia, acute kidney injury, and infection. During the treatment period, she received 120 mg roxadustat orally three times per week. Her HGB level steadily increased from 56 to 151 g/L. After the dosage of roxadustat was reduced to 50 mg three times per week, the HGB level gradually decreased and remained at 132 g/L. In this complicated case, roxadustat exhibited efficacy in treating anemia in a patient with autoimmune disease and infectious complications.

SLE is an autoimmune disease that mainly affects young women and is characterized by circulating antinuclear antibodies that recognize nucleic acids and nucleic acid-binding proteins. Individuals with SLE can have a diverse set of symptoms. Almost any tissue can be the target of autoimmune attack in this disease [1]. Anemia is also common in people with SLE, in whom it can vary from mild to severe. Multiple etiologies contribute to anemia in patients with SLE, including autoimmune hemolytic anemia caused by anti-RBC antibodies, chronic inflammation, and kidney disease [2]. Previous studies have demonstrated that dysregulated innate immune responses and impaired B-cell tolerance lead to a feed-forward loop of innate immune activation, type I interferon secretion, and autoantibody production, all of which can promote anemia in patients with SLE [2, 3]. In addition, LN is the most common form of severe organ damage and the primary cause of death in SLE patients. Severe LN flares can result in acute kidney injury. The use of immunosuppressive agents for the treatment of LN may be accompanied by side effects, including infection and bone marrow hypoplasia. These confounding factors increase the difficulty of treating anemia in SLE patients [2, 4]. In this present case, the results of laboratory tests and bone marrow puncture indicated multiple etiologies of anemia, including chronic inflammation, kidney disease, and bone marrow hypoplasia. In this complicated status, roxadustat showed efficacy in terms of alleviating anemia.

Roxadustat, a representative hypoxia-inducible factor prolyl hydroxylase inhibitor (HIF-PHI), is a new class of oral drug for the treatment of anemia [5]. HIF is a key transcription factor that regulates the expression of hundreds of genes that respond to hypoxia. Thus, HIF-PHIs can affect multiple targets in hypoxia, including EPO from the kidney and/or liver and genes associated with iron absorption and mobilization. Several randomized controlled trials (RCTs) have demonstrated the obvious advantages of HIF-PHIs in non-dialysis CKD and dialysis patients, such as stimulating the HGB response without being influenced by apparent inflammation [5–7]. Recently, a meta-analysis further showed that HIF-PHIs promote iron utilization and maintain the erythropoietic response independent of the inflammatory state [8]. The data from this case revealed decreased ferritin levels, accompanied by increased serum iron and unsaturated iron transferrin saturation levels. These findings suggest the potential of roxadustat for the treatment of anemia in non-dialysis-dependent patients with chronic inflammation.

References

1. Tsokos GC. Autoimmunity and organ damage in systemic lupus erythematosus. Nat Immunol. 2020;21(6):605–14.
2. Giannouli S, Voulgarelis M, Ziakas PD, Tzioufas AG. Anaemia in systemic lupus erythematosus: from pathophysiology to clinical assessment. Ann Rheum Dis. 2006;65(2):144–8.
3. Elkon KB, Wiedeman A. Type I IFN system in the development and manifestations of SLE. Curr Opin Rheumatol. 2012;24(5):499–505.
4. Canny SP, Orozco SL, Thulin NK, Hamerman JA. Immune mechanisms in inflammatory anemia. Annu Rev Immunol. 2023;41:405–29.
5. Chen N, Hao C, Liu BC, et al. Roxadustat treatment for anemia in patients undergoing long-term dialysis. N Engl J Med. 2019;381(11):1011–22.
6. Provenzano R, Shutov E, Eremeeva L, et al. Roxadustat for anemia in patients with end-stage renal disease incident to dialysis. Nephrol Dial Transplant. 2021;36(9):1717–30.

7. Akizawa T, Iwasaki M, Otsuka T, Yamaguchi Y, Reusch M. Phase 3 study of roxadustat to treat anemia in non-dialysis-dependant CKD. Kidney Int Rep. 2021;6(7):1810–28.
8. Zheng Q, Zhang P, Yang H, et al. Effects of hypoxia-inducible factor prolyl hydroxylase inhibitors versus erythropoiesis-stimulating agents on iron metabolism and inflammation in patients undergoing dialysis: a systematic review and meta-analysis. Heliyon. 2023;9(4):e15310.

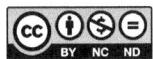

A Case of Cardiorenal Anemia Syndrome Complicated with Malignant Hypertension

22

Xiaoyi Xu, Hong Cheng, and Weijing Bian

22.1 Case Presentation

A 49-year-old male was admitted to our hospital due to hypertension for more than 30 years and intermittent chest tightness for 5 days on December 10, 2020. The patient complained of elevated blood pressure during physical examination more than 30 years ago; blood pressure was not specified, and he did not receive any treatment. Six years prior to admission, he had occasional blood pressure measurements of up to 150–160/100–110 mmHg, without dizziness, headache, blurred vision, or medication. Five days to admission, the patient began to experience chest discomfort and shortness of breath without obvious inducement, which worsened after activities. The patient could fall asleep in the supine position at night without paroxysmal nocturnal dyspnea, edema, or reduced urine output. The patient visited the local hospital, with a blood pressure of 276/165 mmHg, a hemoglobin (Hb) level of 81 g/L, a platelet (PLT) count of 80×10^9/L, a urine protein score of 2+, a red blood cell (RBC) count of 3–6/HPF, a serum creatinine (SCr) of 560 μmol/L, a K+ of 2.72 mmol/L, an albumin (Alb) of 34.1 g/L, a cardiac troponin I (cTnI) of 0.76 ng/mL, a creatine kinase-MB (CK-MB) of 3.98 ng/mL, a myoglobin (Myo) of 209 ng/mL, a brain natriuretic peptide (BNP) of 766 pg/mL, and a lactate dehydrogenase (LDH) of 1003 U/L. He was given antihypertensive and diuretic treatments; his blood pressure decreased to 170–180/100–110 mmHg, and his chest discomfort and shortness of breath resolved. He also reported that nocturia increased over the last 2 months.

He denied any history of diabetes, coronary heart disease, or cerebrovascular disease. He had been smoking for 15 years, smoking an average of 10 cigarettes/day. He did not have a history of alcohol abuse. His father had hypertension; his mother was healthy, and one older brother and two younger brothers also had hypertension.

X. Xu · H. Cheng (✉) · W. Bian
Department of Nephrology, Beijing Anzhen Hospital, Capital Medical University, Beijing, China

© The Author(s) 2025
B.-C. Liu (ed.), *Treatment of Refractory Renal Anemia*,
https://doi.org/10.1007/978-981-97-7636-8_22

Physical examination at admission revealed a temperature of 36.8 °C, a pulse of 104 bpm, a respiratory rate of 20 breaths per minute, and a blood pressure of 168/93 mmHg. His body mass index (BMI) was 25.5 kg/m^2, and his waist circumference was 88 cm. There was no systemic rash or facial edema. Clear breath sounds were noted in both lungs. No dry or wet rales were heard. His heart rate was 104 bpm, in regular rhythm, and no murmur was heard in any of the valve areas. No edema of either lower limb was observed.

Laboratory tests revealed the following results: white blood cell (WBC) count, 5.6 × 10^9/L; Hb, 70 g/L; PLT count, 107 × 10^9/L; routine urine protein, +; routine urine sediment microscopy, 3–7 RBCs/HPF, 0–2 WBCs/HPF, 0–2 granular casts/LPF; urine protein quantification, 1.0 g/d; SCr, 727.5 μmol/L; blood urea nitrogen (BUN), 31.5 mmol/L; urine α1-microblobulin, 86.9 mg/L; biochemistry tests, ALB, 32.8 g/L; globulin (Glo), 23.0 g/L; UA, 632.4 μmol/L; corrected Ca, 2.0 mmol/L; Pi, 1.92 mmol/L; K, 3.09 mmol/L; Cl-, 99.5 mmol/L; intact parathyroid hormone (iPTH), 436.1 pg/mL; LDH, 701 U/L; high-sensitivity troponin I (hsTnI), 824.5 pg/mL; CK-MB, 1.4 ng/mL; Myo, 158.9 ng/mL; BNP, 366 pg/mL; N-terminal pro b-type natriuretic peptide (NT-proBNP), 17,502 pg/mL; high-sensitivity C-reactive protein (hsCRP), >20 mg/L; serum ferritin (SF), 755 ng/mL; and transferrin saturation (TSAT), 25.2%.

Immune-related tests revealed negative anti-nuclear antibody (ANA), anti-double-stranded DNA (anti-ds-DNA) antibody, and anti-extractable nuclear antigen (anti-ENA) profiles; immunoglobulins, including IgA, IgG, IgM, and complement, were all normal; test results for antineutrophil cytoplasmic antibody (ANCA) and anti-glomerular basement membrane (anti-GBM) antibodies were negative; furthermore, peripheral blood smears revealed fragmented RBCs (Fig. 22.1).

Abdominal ultrasound revealed a left kidney measuring 10.3 × 5.8 × 5.0 cm, with a parenchymal thickness of 1.4 cm; a right kidney measuring 10.8 × 4.7 × 4.1 cm, with a parenchymal thickness of 1.2 cm; and poor structure in both kidneys. Echocardiography revealed a left ventricular ejection fraction (LVEF) of 63%, a left

Fig. 22.1 Peripheral blood smear showing fragmented red blood cells (red arrows)

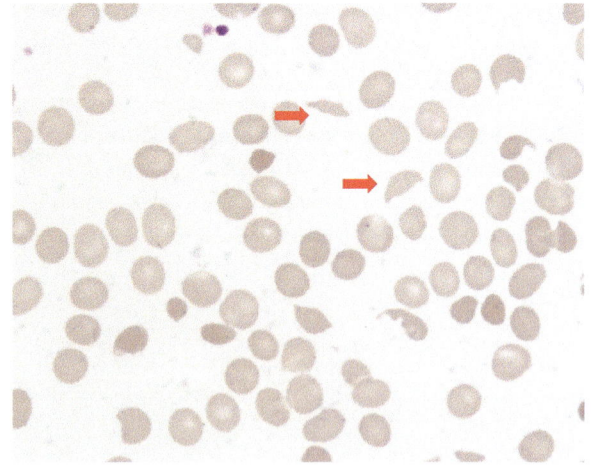

ventricular posterior wall of 12 mm, an interventricular septum of 13 mm, a left ventricular end diastolic diameter (LVEDd) of 53 mm, a left atrium (LA) of $40 \times 50 \times 51$ mm, and abnormal segmental wall motion. Carotid ultrasound revealed bilateral carotid plaques, mainly on the left side. Fundus examination revealed scattered retinal hemorrhage and exudation, and papilledema was observed. No significant stenosis was observed at the initial segment of both renal arteries during renal artery ultrasound. An adrenal gland computed tomography (CT) scan did not reveal any significant abnormalities. His coronary artery calcium score was 270.4, indicating moderate coronary artery calcium. Abdominal X-ray did not show obvious abdominal aortic calcification.

The patient was a middle-aged male, and although elevated SCr was found for only 3 days and his urine output was not reduced, he had nocturia, and he showed poor structure of both kidneys on ultrasound, which suggests chronic renal insufficiency. Because the patient had a quantitative urine protein concentration of 1 g/d and minimal microscopic hematuria, as well as a more than 30-year history of hypertension without treatment, preexisting hypertensive retinopathy, and hypertensive cardiac changes, hypertensive renal injury was considered the major etiology of chronic renal insufficiency. This medical visit was due to an acute exacerbation of chronic kidney disease. At the time of this episode in the local hospital, his blood pressure was 276/165 mmHg, which remained as high as 170–180/100–110 mmHg after therapy, and there was papilledema; thus, the diagnosis of malignant hypertension was confirmed. At the same time, the patient had anemia, thrombocytopenia, elevated LDH, and fragmented RBCs that were easily observed in the peripheral blood, suggesting the presence of microangiopathic hemolytic anemia. Malignant hypertension leading to thrombotic microangiopathy was considered, which in turn predisposed the patient to acute kidney injury based on chronic renal insufficiency. Moreover, the patient had a prominent loss of activity tolerance, chest tightness, and shortness of breath during the disease course. BNP and NT-proBNP were significantly increased, indicating the presence of acute heart failure. Heart failure, acute kidney injury, and anemia aggravated one another and continued to worsen, leading to cardiorenal anemia syndrome. In summary, the final diagnosis of this patient was as follows:

1. Chronic renal failure: renal anemia, chronic kidney disease-mineral and bone disorder (CKD-MBD), hyperphosphatemia, secondary hyperparathyroidism, and coronary artery calcification (moderate).
2. Acute kidney injury (probable): thrombotic microangiopathy (probable), type 1 cardiorenal syndrome.
3. Acute heart failure: cardiac function class III (New York Heart Association [NYHA] classification).
4. Malignant hypertension.
5. Hypertensive renal impairment (probable): hypertensive retinopathy.

It is necessary to break the vicious cycle of acute kidney injury, anemia, and acute heart injury in patients with cardiorenal anemia syndrome. Moreover, multiple

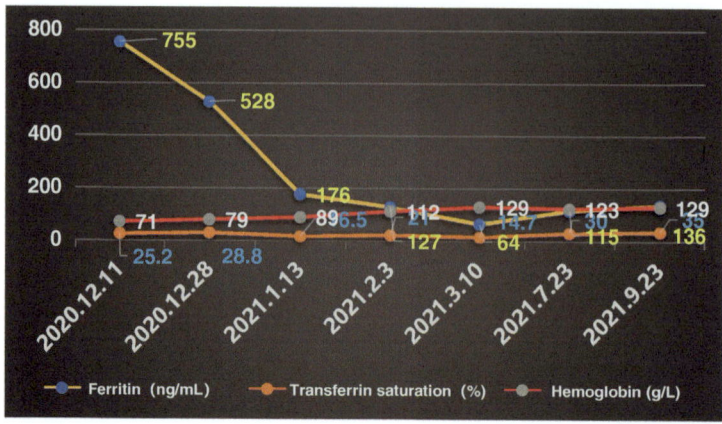

Fig. 22.2 Changes in hemoglobin and iron parameters after treatment

cardiorenal multidisciplinary team (MDT) interventions were administered to the patient. He was given sacubitril/valsartan 50 mg bid (titration to 100 mg bid later), benidipine 4 mg bid, arotinolol hydrochloride 10 mg bid, and torsemide 5 mg qd to control blood pressure and treat heart failure. He was subsequently *treated with bayaspirin and atorvastatin*. For chronic renal insufficiency, the patient was given compound α-ketoacid, Bailing Capsule, and Niaoduqing, while CKD-MBD was treated with sevelamer carbonate; roxadustat and ferrous succinate were given for renal anemia.

After the MDT treatments mentioned earlier, the symptoms of chest discomfort and shortness of breath were relieved; activity tolerance increased, and blood pressure was controlled at 130–140/70–80 mmHg. The changes in laboratory test results were as follows: Hb 71 g/L → 129 g/L, SF 755 ng/mL → 136 ng/mL, TSAT 25% → 35% (Fig. 22.2), BNP 766 pg/mL → 88 pg/mL, NT-proBNP 6998 pg/mL → 266 pg/mL, SCr 797 μmol/L → 170-190 μmol/L, PLT 70 × 10⁹/L → 178 × 10⁹/L, LDH 698 U/L → 182 U/L, and serum potassium was essentially normal. From December 2020 to April and September 2021, the LVEF increased from 63% to 65% and 75%, respectively, and the pulmonary artery pressure decreased from 45 mmHg to 29 mmHg and 25 mmHg.

22.2   Discussion

This is a middle-aged male patient diagnosed with malignant hypertension complicated by cardiorenal anemia syndrome.

Oxidative stress, inflammation, and renin-angiotensin system activation are all pathogenic mechanisms of cardiorenal syndrome. However, the pathogenesis of cardiorenal anemia syndrome is more complicated, and CKD may further exacerbate cardiac injury due to relatively low erythropoietin (EPO) and decreased Hb levels. Anemia causes a decrease in blood viscosity, increases venous return, and increases cardiac compensatory efforts in patients with cardiovascular disease (CVD); it also worsens heart failure and promotes worsening disease progression in CKD patients. The inflammatory state in CVD and CKD patients may also aggravate anemia, leading to increased mortality in patients with a poor prognosis [1]. Therefore, the treatment of cardiorenal anemia syndrome must involve comprehensive management of multiple targets, and overcoming the "death triangle," i.e., anemia, CKD, and CVD, is crucial.

Correction of anemia in this patient with cardiorenal anemia syndrome began from many aspects, such as controlling blood pressure, improving cardiac function, and correcting anemia. The pathogenesis of renal anemia mainly includes various factors, including EPO deficiency, iron metabolism disorders, and inflammation [2]. Roxadustat is a hypoxia-inducible factor-prolyl hydroxylase inhibitor (HIF-PHI) that acts by inhibiting prolyl hydroxylase, stabilizing the HIF pathway, regulating iron metabolism, upregulating iron absorption/transport-related gene expression, and inhibiting hepcidin, which comprehensively regulates erythropoiesis [2, 3]. A phase 3 clinical study in China showed that, in anemic patients with nondialysis CKD, roxadustat was effective in correcting anemia and increasing iron utilization without the need for routine intravenous iron supplementation [4]; in patients with CKD-induced anemia on dialysis, the efficacy of anemia correction was comparable in the roxadustat group compared with the erythropoiesis-stimulating agent (ESA) group, without the need for routine intravenous iron supplementation, and was not influenced by the inflammatory status of the patients. In conclusion, roxadustat has several advantages for anemia correction in patients with cardiorenal anemia syndrome [5].

The CHOIR study showed a significantly increased risk of composite endpoint events (death, myocardial infarction, hospitalization for congestive heart failure, and stroke) in patients with nondialysis renal anemia with increasing recombinant human erythropoietin (rHuEPO) doses, independent of Hb levels [6]. In addition, the patient in our case had a long history of hypertension, which had not been previously treated. His blood pressure reached 276/165 mmHg during this episode, and he was diagnosed with malignant hypertension. Hypertension is a common complication of ESA treatment. Studies have shown that switching medications from ESA to roxadustat in patients undergoing peritoneal dialysis is effective in preventing ESA-related increases in blood pressure [7].

Based on the abovementioned findings, we treated this patient with roxadustat for anemia while improving iron metabolism in the inflammatory state, and we observed that the patient had decreased serum ferritin levels and increased iron saturation levels, which is consistent with the findings of previous clinical studies of roxadustat. In addition, after simultaneous antihypertensive and diuretic treatment, the patient's blood pressure stabilized, and his cardiac function also improved.

References

1. Tanaka T, Eckardt KU. HIF activation against CVD in CKD: novel treatment opportunities. Semin Nephrol. 2018;38(3):267–76.
2. Koury MJ, Haase VH. Anaemia in kidney disease: harnessing hypoxia responses for therapy. Nat Rev Nephrol. 2015;11(7):394–410.

3. Knutson MD. Iron transport proteins: gateways of cellular and systemic iron homeostasis. J Biol Chem. 2017;292(31):12735–43.
4. Chen N, Hao C, Peng X, et al. Roxadustat for anemia in patients with kidney disease not receiving dialysis. N Engl J Med. 2019;381(11):1001–10.
5. Chen N, Hao C, Liu BC, et al. Roxadustat treatment for anemia in patients undergoing long-term dialysis. N Engl J Med. 2019;381(11):1011–22.
6. Singh AK, Szczech L, Tang KL, et al. Correction of anemia with epoetin alfa in chronic kidney disease. N Engl J Med. 2006;355(20):2085–98.
7. Zhao YC, Zhao HP, Wu B, et al. Effect of roxostat on blood pressure in maintenance peritoneal dialysis patients. Chin J Blood Purif. 2022;21(9):633–7.

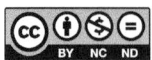

Roxadustat Quickly Corrected Anemia in a Peritoneal Dialysis Patient and Increased Perioperative Safety

Xin-Wang Zhu and Li Yao

23.1 Case Presentation

A 27-year-old female patient was admitted due to an increase in serum creatinine levels for 3.5 years, peritoneal dialysis (PD) for more than 1 month, and catheter outflow dysfunction for 2 days on April 28, 2021.

The patient had taken traditional Chinese medicine orally for 1 month due to irregular menstruation 3.5 years prior to admission and then found an elevated serum creatinine level of 140 μmol/L. She was then diagnosed with tubulointerstitial nephropathy (drug induced likely) and chronic renal insufficiency (stage G3b) according to renal biopsy findings. She was given prednisone acetate, Haikun Shenxi and Shenkangning (traditional Chinese medicine compound preparation), α-ketoacid tablets, and calcium dobesilate to improve renal function, which was supplemented with antianemia therapy and acid-inhibiting agents. Her serum creatinine (Scr) level was 130 μmol/L before discharge. One month prior to admission, the patient returned to our hospital for further examination. Urine analysis revealed a large amount of mixed proteinuria, Scr level of 1486 μmol/L, and hemoglobin (Hb) concentration of 55 g/L. After right internal jugular vein catheterization, hemodialysis treatment was started three times a week. She underwent peritoneal dialysis(PD) catheterization in our department on March 11, 2021, and PD treatment began after surgery. The PD regimen was 2000 mL of 1.5% PD solution, 3 times in the day, 3 h in each dwell, and 2000 ml of 2.5% PD solution, 11 h at night, and the ultrafiltration volume was approximately 400 ml. Two days prior to admission, the catheter outflow drainage was not smooth, but no abdominal pain or cloudy dialysis effluent were noted. Her urine volume at that time was approximately 1300–1800 mL/day, with edema of the eyelids and both lower limbs. There was no significant change in her body weight.

X.-W. Zhu · L. Yao (✉)
Department of Nephrology, The First Hospital of China Medical University, Shenyang, China

© The Author(s) 2025
B.-C. Liu (ed.), *Treatment of Refractory Renal Anemia*,
https://doi.org/10.1007/978-981-97-7636-8_23

The patient had a more than 1-month history of hypertension, and blood pressure (BP) reached 160/110 mmHg. At the time of admission, the patient was taking 30 mg of nifedipine (Adalat) once orally, and her blood pressure was controlled at approximately 145/100 mmHg. On February 27, 2021, 4 units of blood was transfused cumulatively at another hospital. The patient had a 2-month history of neovascular glaucoma in the left eye, central retinal vein occlusion in the left eye, and uveitis in the left eye and a 1-month history of postoperative vitrectomy in the left eye and aphakia in the left eye for 1 month. There was no menorrhagia.

Physical examination revealed BP of 130/92 mmHg, and her eyelids were edematous; her conjunctiva was pale, and her lips and nail beds were pale. The abdomen was flat and soft without tenderness; there was no abdominal muscle tension. There was mild pitting edema in both lower extremities. The scar from PD catheterization was observed 2 cm to the left of the midline of the abdomen. One PD catheter was observed on the abdominal wall. There was no obvious redness or swelling at the catheter exit site or exudation.

Laboratory examinations revealed the following: white blood cell (WBC) count, 3.40×10^9/L; red blood cell (RBC) count, 2.39×10^{12}/L; Hb, 66 g/L; hematocrit (HCT), 0.199; platelet (PLT) count, 104×10^9/L, total protein, 55.3 g/L; albumin, 33.5 g/L; urea, 15.82 mmol/L; creatinine (Cr), 1009 μmol/L(reference range, 58–110 μmol/L); serum potassium, 4.58 mmol/L; serum calcium, 2.35 mmol/L; phosphorus, 1.17 mmol/L; estimated glomerular filtration rate (eGFR), 4.1; C-reactive protein, 2.50 mg/L; and procalcitonin, 0.218 ng/mL. Coagulation function parameters were as follows: prothrombin time, 13.7 s; activated partial thromboplastin time, 36.9 s; fibrinogen, 3.23 g/L; D-dimer, 0.28 μg/mL; and brain natriuretic peptide, 151 pg/mL. The result of fecal occult blood test was negative.

Ultrasonography of the liver, gallbladder, spleen, and pancreas revealed echogenic changes in both kidneys, consistent with chronic renal damage and bilateral renal cysts. In echocardiography, the volume of the left atrium was slightly greater; the overall systolic function of the left ventricle was normal at rest, and the ejection fraction was 60%. On whole-abdominal computed tomography (CT), the outlines of both kidneys were irregular, and the local renal parenchyma was slightly thinner. Multiple small cysts were observed in the left kidney. The left adrenal gland was thickened. The retroperitoneal lymph nodes were enlarged.

23.2 Diagnosis

PD catheter dysfunction (most likely due to omental wrapping).

Chronic renal insufficiency (G5D, PD stage), renal anemia, chronic kidney disease-mineral bone disorder (CKD-MBD), metabolic acidosis.

Chronic interstitial nephritis.

Hypertension grade 2 (very high risk).

Neovascular glaucoma, central retinal vein occlusion, uveitis in the left eye.

For PD, pelvic X-ray revealed a normal position of the PD catheter (Fig. 23.1). During peritoneal washing or PD treatment, the PD solution could not be drained,

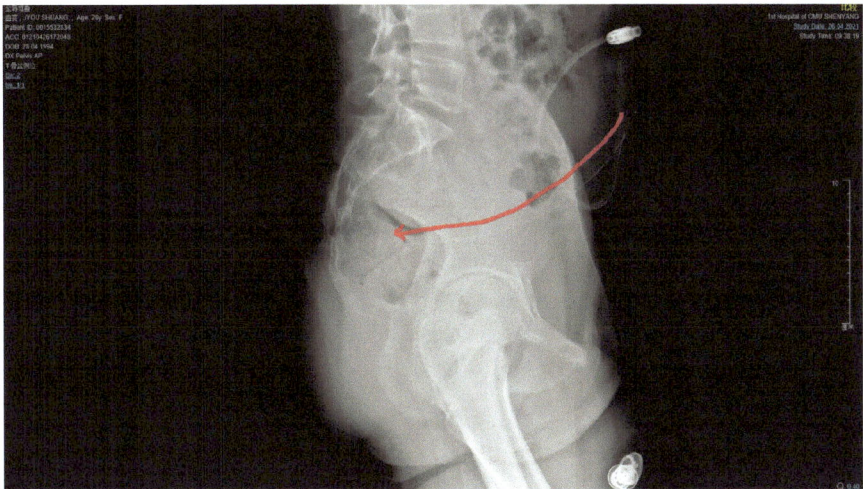

Fig. 23.1 On April 29, 2021, reexamination of the pelvis was performed due to catheter outflow dysfunction. X-ray revealed that the tip position of the PD catheter was in the pelvis. The patient had fluid flow restriction. Omental wrapping or obstruction by other adherent intraperitoneal tissues was considered

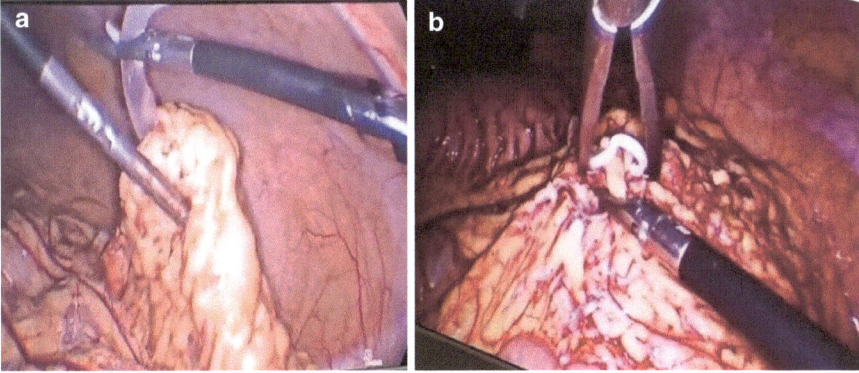

Fig. 23.2 Laparoscopic surgery under general anesthesia. (**a**) The PD catheter is occluded by the greater omentum. (**b**) After releasing the wrapped PD catheter, the greater omentum was suspended with a Hemolock clip, and then the PD catheter was fixed on the inner abdominal wall using No. 7 silk thread

but there was no obvious resistance when the PD solution was injected into the peritoneal cavity through the catheter. However, there was no improvement after the interventions, such as urokinase sealing or radiological manipulation. Surgical treatment was recommended to relieve the omental wrapping. On April 29, laparoscopic adhesiolysis and greater omentum folding were performed, and then PD catheter internal fixation was performed under general anesthesia, as shown in Fig. 23.2. Postoperative PD fluid drainage was unobstructed, but the effluent was pale and bloody (see Fig. 23.3). Low-dose tidal peritoneal dialysis (TPD) therapy was initiated.

For renal anemia, recombinant human erythropoietin (r-HuEPO，3000 IU) was regularly injected subcutaneously three times a week before the operation; 150 mg of polysaccharide-iron complex was taken two times a day orally, and 15 ml of Shengxuebao Mixture was taken three times a day orally. Considering that the patient had low response to conventional dose of EPO, and laparoscopic intraoperative bleeding and postoperative bloody peritoneal dialysate would further aggravate anemia, the patient's medication was switched to roxadustat at a dosage of 100 mg three times per week (patient weight, 50 kg). The patient's Hb increased rapidly (Fig. 23.4) and avoided transfusion again. The anemia-related parameters before and after roxadustat administration are shown in Table 23.1.

Other treatments include calcitriol capsules (0.25 µg once a day orally), calcium carbonate D3 granules (500 mg once a day orally with meals), and nifedipine (30 mg once a day orally).

Fig. 23.3 Postoperative abdominal bleeding

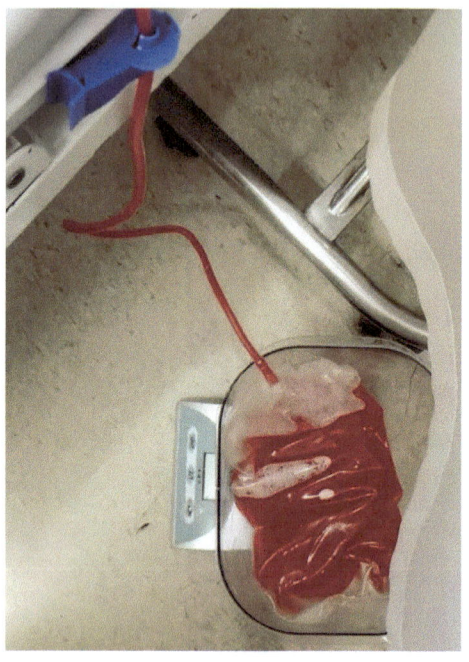

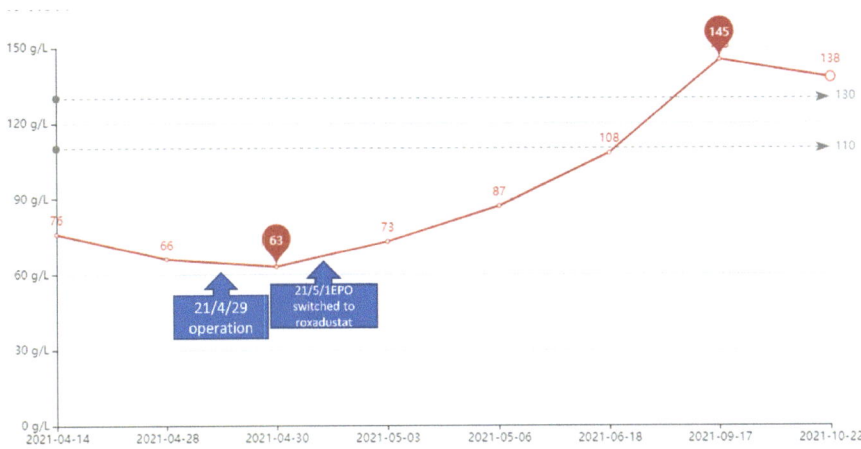

Fig. 23.4 Perioperative anti-anemia treatment and changes in Hb levels

Table 23.1 Changes of anemia and iron storage before and after treatment

	Item	Unit	Normal range	Before medication	After medication	
				21/4/29	2021/5/6
Blood routine examination	Hemoglobin，Hb	g/L	130–175	66	87
	Red blood cell count, RBC	10^12/L	4.3–5.8	2.39	3.27
	Hematocrit, HCT	L/L	0.4–0.5	0.199	0.269
	Mean corpuscular volume, MCV	fL	82–100	83.3	82.3
	Mean corpuscular hemoglobin content, HCT	Pg	27–34	27.6	26.6
	Mean corpuscular-hemoglobin concentration, MCHC	g/L	316–354	332	323
	White blood cell count, WBC	10^9/L	3.5–9.5	3.4	4.67
	Neutrophil count, NE#	10^9/L	1.8–6.3	1.91	2.79
	Blood platelet count, PLT	10^9/L	125–350	104	170
Iron store	Serum iron, Fe	µmol/L	8.1–28.3	9.1	6
	Transferrin, TRF	Mg/dL	200–360	223	207
	Transferrin saturation, TSAT	%	>20%	16.24%	11.54%
	Ferritin, Fer	µg/L	30–400	103	28
	Folate	Nmol/L	8.83–60.8	10.6	6.58
	Vitamin B12, VB12	Pmol/L	145–637	303	185

23.3 Discussion

Before hospitalization, a regular dose of EPO supplement was given, but the patient seemed unresponsive. However, the patient experienced intra-abdominal bleeding after laparoscopic surgery; the effluent was bloody, and Hb continued to decrease. The patient is preparing for kidney transplantation; therefore, blood transfusions were avoided as much as possible to reduce the risk of future kidney transplant rejection. On May 1, 2021, 100 mg of roxadustat was added orally three times a week. The Hb was noted to increase from 63 to 87 g/L in less than 1 week, showing that roxadustat could quickly relieve renal anemia, shorten the length of hospital stay, and reduce the need for blood transfusion. While roxadustat rapidly corrected renal anemia, serum iron, ferritin, and other parameters decreased, indicating that the rapid correction of anemia accelerated the consumption of iron and that hematopoietic raw material supplementation should continue to be provided (Table 23.1).

At present, the standard treatment for renal anemia is erythropoietin (EPO) replacement therapy, but the effects on inflammatory status, blood pressure, serum potassium, and other factors should be considered when EPO is used and the increase in Hb is not significant or Hb even continues to decrease in the early stage of treatment [1]. Roxadustat affects various hematopoietic stages, such as iron absorption, iron utilization, the promotion of endogenous EPO production, and the enhancement of receptor sensitivity and can rapidly increase Hb levels in PD patients [2]. This approach can help correct anemia in perioperative patients as soon as possible, reduce the need for blood transfusion, increase surgical safety, and shorten postoperative recovery time and hospital stay.

References

1. Chen N, Hao C, Liu BC, et al. Roxadustat treatment for anemia in patients undergoing long-term dialysis. N Engl J Med. 2019;381(11):1011–22.
2. Zhu XW, Zhang CX, Xu TH, et al. Therapeutic effect of roxalrestat on 29 cases of renal anemia in peritoneal dialysis. Chin J Prac Inter Med. 2020;40(11):932–6.

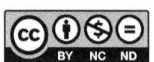

Treatment of Refractory Anemia in a Patient with End-Stage Renal Disease and a Postoperative Bladder Tumor

Nan Zhu, Pei Wang, and Zhangsuo Liu

24.1 Case Presentation

A 72-year-old man was admitted with the chief complaint of "discovered renal function abnormalities for more than 2 years, regular hemodialysis for more than 6 months, and weakness for 1 week." More than 2 years ago, the patient had gross hematuria with no obvious cause, without urinary frequency, urgency, pain, or difficulty in urination. His laboratory examination showed the following: urine occult blood test, 3+; blood urea nitrogen, 13.9 mmol/L; serum creatinine, 210 μmol/L; and serum uric acid, 469 μmol/L. Color Doppler ultrasound showed multiple bladder masses. Then, he visited the department of urology of our hospital for "transurethral bladder tumor resection" (Fig. 24.1). Over 6 months earlier, the patient returned to the department of urology for reexamination due to poor appetite and chest tightness. His laboratory examinations revealed the following: hemoglobin, 98 g/L; serum potassium, 5.53 mmol/L; serum calcium, 2.08 mmol/L; phosphorus, 1.6 mmol/L; blood urea nitrogen, 38.4 mmol/L; serum creatinine, 851 μmol/L; and NT-proBNP 20,087 pg/mL. The patient was then diagnosed with (1) chronic kidney disease (stage 5) with renal anemia and hyperkalemia, (2) heart failure, (3) hypertension, (4) type 2 diabetes, and (5) postoperative bladder tumor. He was initially treated with hemodialysis thrice weekly after an arteriovenous fistula was established. He received intravenous recombinant human erythropoietin (r-HuEPO) at a dose of 8000 U/week to treat anemia, as well as management procedures for high blood pressure and hyperglycemia.

N. Zhu · P. Wang (✉)
Blood Purification Center, The First Affiliated Hospital of Zhengzhou University, Zhengzhou, China

Z. Liu (✉)
Blood Purification Center, The First Affiliated Hospital of Zhengzhou University, Zhengzhou, China

Henan Province Research Center for Kidney Disease, Zhengzhou, China

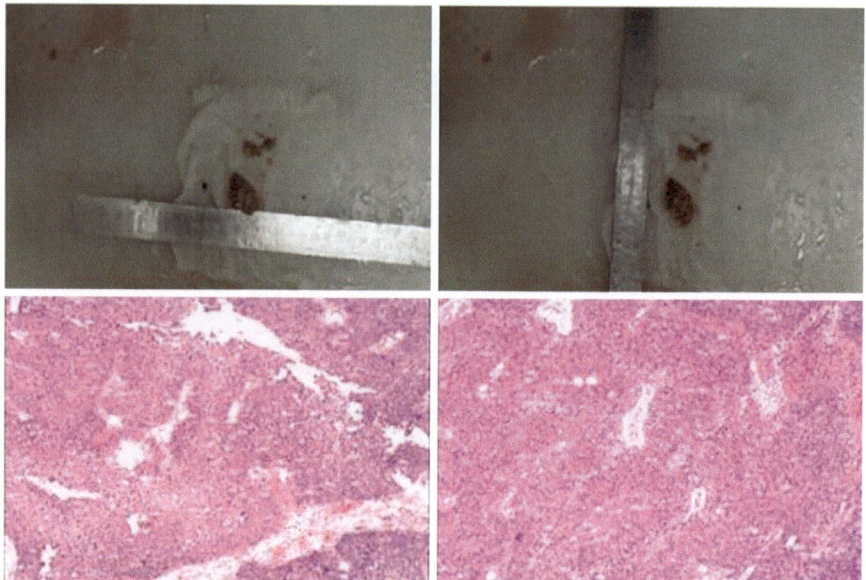

Fig. 24.1 Invasive papillary urothelial carcinoma, high-grade

The patient had over 20-year history of diabetes for which he was treated with recombinant human insulin at a dose of 16 IU in the morning and 14 IU in the evening. He also had a history of hypertension for 20 years, with a highest blood pressure of 190/90 mmHg, and was currently treated with sacubitril/valsartan, nifedipine sustained-release tablets, and terazosin hydrochloride tablets, achieving blood pressure control at 150–160/80–90 mmHg. He underwent transurethral bladder tumor resection in our hospital in December 2017, March 2018, and July 2018, and no metastases were found. He had a history of coronary heart disease for 3 months that was being treated with enteric-coated aspirin and clopidogrel sulfate tablets. He denied any other significant personal or family medical history. Physical examination showed a height of 175 cm, weight of 65 kg, blood pressure of 162/83 mmHg, heart rate of 84 beats/min, mild pitting edema in both lower limbs, no obvious abnormalities in heart and lung auscultation, anemic appearance, and pale skin and mucous membranes.

Laboratory examinations revealed the following: hemoglobin, 86 g/L; hematocrit, 0.30; ferritin, 1579.1 ng/ml; transferrin saturation, 92%; hepcidin, 104.15 ng/mL; folic acid, 23 ng/mL; vitamin B12, 288 pg/mL; serum potassium, 6.38 mmol/L; serum calcium, 2.25 mmol/L; phosphorus, 1.17 mmol/L; albumin, 38.7 g/L; alkaline phosphatase, 68 U/L; blood urea nitrogen, 21.4 mmol/L; serum creatinine, 719 μmol/L; total cholesterol, 3.83 mmol/L; triglyceride, 1.17 mmol/L; iPTH, 128 pg/mL; Nt-proBNP, 2218 pg/ml; C-reactive protein (CRP), 71.58 mg/L; fecal occult blood test, (−); and Coombs test, (−). No obvious abnormalities were found in the liver, gallbladder, pancreas, or spleen by ultrasound.

Preliminary laboratory examinations indicated that the patient had anemia, hyperkalemia, and high levels of ferritin and hepcidin. We provided a comprehensive management for the patient as follows: First, we improved dialysis adequacy by increasing blood flow and changing the dialyzer, to achieve a spKt/v of 1.5–1.7. Second, to manage hyperkalemia, we strengthened nutritional education and modified his diet plan to avoid high-potassium foods and recommended foods with lower phosphorus/protein. Third, for his anemia, we investigated the common causes of anemia. This patient had no excessive loss of red blood cells, such as gastrointestinal bleeding, and there was no hemolytic anemia or hypersplenism. Vitamin B12 and folic acid were within the normal ranges. However, the patient is currently in an inflammatory state with high levels of ferritin and hepcidin and unstable blood pressure, as well as a postoperative tumor. Roxadustat can effectively increase hemoglobin levels without being affected by mild inflammation and can also downregulate ferritin levels, improve various iron metabolism indicators, increase iron utilization, and promote good oral compliance. We prescribed roxadustat orally to correct his anemia. Based on the patient's body weight, an initial dose of 120 mg TIW roxadustat was prescribed. A routine blood examination was performed on December 25, 2019, at which his hemoglobin had decreased from the original 86 g/L to 78.3 g/L. Considering the patient's age and history of cardiovascular disease, a maintenance dose was prescribed. On January 10, 2020, a follow-up examination showed that the hemoglobin level had increased from 78.3 g/L to 94.4 g/L. Thus, the original dose was continued. As of February 17, 2020, the hemoglobin level had increased to 108 g/L; ferritin had reached 1323.4 ng/ml; transferrin saturation had reached 87%, and hepcidin had reached 87.42 ng/mL. The patient was given a reduced dose of 100 mg TIW of roxadustat from February 2020 to July 2020. The hemoglobin concentrations ranged from 110 to 120 g/L. With the improvement of the patient's diet and dialysis quality, the hemoglobin level was rechecked on October 2, 2020, and it was 131 g/L. At this time, the patient stopped taking the medication on his own. His hemoglobin level was 124 g/L on December 7, 2020 and 107 g/L on February 9, 2021. After readministering a dose of 70 mg TIW of roxadustat, the hemoglobin showed 111 g/L on May 12, 2021; ferritin decreased to 623.3 ng/ml, and hepcidin decreased to 10.76 ng/mL. No iron supplements were used during roxadustat treatment, and the changes in hemoglobin are shown in Fig. 24.2. The patient had good overall safety and tolerability and did not experience any adverse reactions, such as nausea, vomiting, or diarrhea. Considering the numerous comorbidities of the patient, we actively provided corresponding treatments for his CKD-MBD, SHPT, and coronary heart disease, as well as hypertension and hyperglycemia. Regular cystoscopy revealed no recurrence or metastasis of tumors (Fig. 24.3).

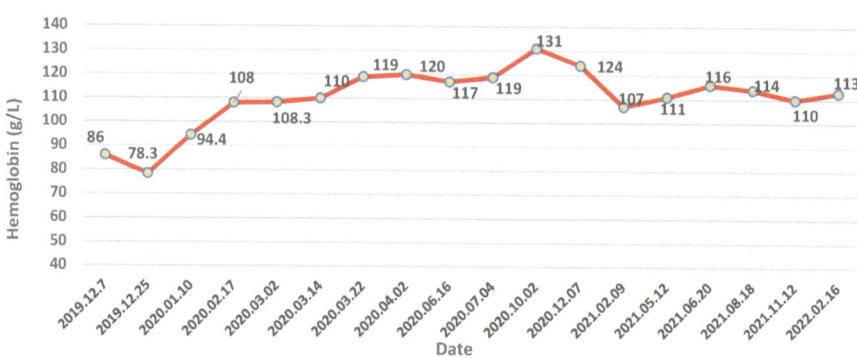

Fig. 24.2 Changes in hemoglobin levels during treatment with roxadustat

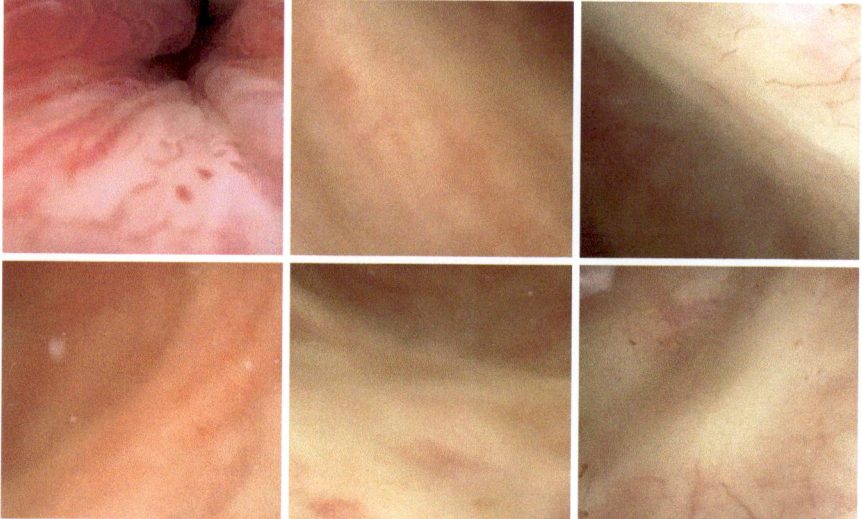

Fig. 24.3 Postoperative changes in bladder tumor, no other obvious abnormalities were observed

24.2 Discussion

As a common complication in hemodialysis patients, renal anemia has the following characteristics: high prevalence, high intervention rate, but low attainment rate [1]. During the past 30 years, erythropoiesis-stimulating agents (ESAs) and iron supplementary agents have been the mainstay of renal anemia treatment [2]. According to the data of the National Blood Purification Case Information Registration System in 2018, ESA usage rate among China's hemodialysis patients was as high as 98.7%. However, the overall hemoglobin target attainment rate for patients was relatively low, with only 37.7% of patients having their hemoglobin levels above 110 g/L. As the causes of anemia are complex, including insufficient EPO production, reduced EPO activity, iron deficiency, metabolic disorders, malnutrition, inflammatory state, uremic toxin, and so on [3], many treatments have limited effectiveness. Additionally, hemodialysis patients often have multiple comorbidities, making the treatment of renal anemia more challenging. Anemia can also increase the risk of cardiovascular events, hospitalization, and death, as well as adding to the economic burden on patients [4]. In our case report, the patient was an elderly male with diabetic nephropathy as the primary disease. He is currently on maintenance hemodialysis and has comorbidities such as hypertension, coronary heart disease, and chronic inflammation. The poor outcomes of ESA treatment in this patient may have resulted from multiple factors, including an inadequate EPO dose, chronic inflammation, malnutrition, and inadequate dialysis. Patients with hyporesponsiveness require a higher dose of ESAs. Considering that high-dose ESA treatment may increase the risk of cardiovascular and cerebrovascular events such as thrombosis, hypertension, and stroke [5, 6], new strategies are therefore needed to reduce these side effects.

Roxadustat (FG-4592), as a new oral medication to treat renal anemia, is a prolyl hydroxylase inhibitor that increases HIF transcriptional activity by stabilizing HIF-α subunits. Increased transcriptional activity can promote erythropoiesis by increasing endogenous EPO [7]. Multiple trials have demonstrated that roxadustat is no less effective than ESAs in patients undergoing hemodialysis [8]. And at the same time, roxadustat can promote the expression of proteins related to iron metabolism and thus reduce hepcidin levels. Compared to ESAs, it can reduce the impact of micro-inflammation on the efficacy of hemoglobin [9, 10]. Thus, the treatment for anemia was switched to roxadustat. After roxadustat treatment, the patient's hemoglobin increased, and his iron metabolism significantly improved. At the same time, the patient's compliance was good. Additionally, drug interactions should be considered, and the timing and dosage of treatment with other drugs should be adjusted in a timely manner. For example, considering that coadministration of sevelamer and roxadustat reduces the blood concentration of roxadustat, the medication time was staggered during use [5].

Meanwhile, studies have shown that high-dose ESA therapy may increase the risk of tumor growth [5, 6], while high-dose intravenous iron agent application may induce severe allergic reactions, iron overload, oxidative stress, cardiovascular disease, and infection [11]. The joint guidelines of the American Society of Clinical Oncology and the American Society of Hematology suggest that unacceptable risks associated with the use of ESAs may outweigh the potential benefits for patients with curable malignancies and those with malignancies who are expected to achieve medium- to long-term survival after chemotherapy; therefore, the guidelines recommend that ESA treatment should be used with caution in patients with malignancies in certain circumstances [5, 12]. The 2012 Kidney Disease Improving Global Outcomes (KDIGO) clinical practice guidelines for anemia also note that ESAs should be used with caution in patients with active malignancy or a history of malignancy [13]. This is also one of the reasons we are considering adjusting from erythropoietin to roxadustat. A global phase III clinical research analysis reveals that both the roxadustat and darbepoetin groups exhibit comparable treatment-emergent adverse events (TEAEs) [14]. In animal models, long-term use of FG-4592 (roxadustat) for up to 2 years in CD-1 mice and Sprague Dawley rats did not increase the risk of tumors [15, 16]. Also, an open-label, phase 2 study of roxadustat for the treatment of anemia in patients receiving chemotherapy for non-myeloid malignancies shows that roxadustat can increase hemoglobin levels in cancer patients with chemotherapy-induced anemia, regardless of the patients' CRP levels [17]. Based on the guidelines, considering the patient's history of bladder tumor surgery, roxadustat was used, and a favorable outcome was achieved for this patient. During the follow-up, no recurrence or metastasis of the tumor was found, and the safety profile was good.

In conclusion, anemia, which is a prevalent and serious complication associated with CKD, may increase the risk of hospitalization and mortality, particularly in end-stage renal disease (ESRD) patients undergoing hemodialysis [4]. The traditional treatment of renal anemia includes iron agents, ESAs, and RBC transfusion [2]. ESAs are the analogs of EPO with characteristics of good tolerance and ease to use. They have been used to treat anemia patients with normal physiology and can significantly improve the quality of life of patients. However, ESAs can increase blood pressure, promote tumor growth, and increase the risk of stroke and thromboembolism in patients with malignant tumors [5, 6]. Meanwhile, HIF-PHI could promote the expression of iron metabolism-related proteins by promoting EPO production and its receptor expression and reducing hepcidin levels, thereby comprehensively regulating the production of erythrocytes [7–10]. Roxadustat was officially approved by the State Drug Administration of China to treat CKD anemia in dialysis patients, but it has not been used to treat cancer-related anemia. Since our report is just an individual case, more clinical trials are needed to observe the therapeutic effect and mechanism of roxadustat for anemia treatment in cancer patients with ESRD.

References

1. Zhou QG, Jiang JP, Wu SJ, et al. Current pattern of Chinese dialysis units: a cohort study in a representative sample of units. Chin Med J. 2012;125(19):3434–9.
2. Johnson DW, Pollock CA, Macdougall IC. Erythropoiesis-stimulating agent hyporesponsiveness. Nephrology. 2007;12(4):321–30.
3. Liu J, Yang F, Waheed Y, et al. The role of roxadustat in chronic kidney disease patients complicated with anemia. Korean J Intern Med. 2023;38(2):147–56.
4. Thorp ML, Johnson ES, Yang X, et al. Effect of anaemia on mortality, cardiovascular hospitalizations and end-stage renal disease among patients with chronic kidney disease. Nephrology (Carlton). 2009;14(2):240–6.
5. Nephrology Physicians Branch of Chinese Medical Doctor Association Nephrology Guidelines Working Group. Clinical practice guidelines for the diagnosis and treatment of renal anemia in China. Chin Med J. 2021;101(20):1463–502.
6. Koulouridis I, Alfayez M, Trikalinos TA, et al. Dose of erythropoiesis-stimulating agents and adverse outcomes in CKD: a metaregression analysis. Am J Kidney Dis. 2013;61(1):44–56.
7. Becker K, Saad M. A new approach to the management of anemia in CKD patients: a review on roxadustat. Adv Ther. 2017;34(4):848–53.
8. Chen N, Hao C, Liu B-C, et al. Roxadustat treatment for anemia in patients undergoing long-term dialysis. N Engl J Med. 2019;381(11):1011–22.

9. Locatelli F, Del Vecchio L, De Nicola L, et al. Are all erythropoiesis-stimulating agents created equal? Nephrol Dial Transplant. 2021;36(8):1369–77.

10. Maxwell PH, Eckardt KU. HIF prolyl hydroxylase inhibitors for the treatment of renal anaemia and beyond. Nat Rev Nephrol. 2016;12(3):157–68.

11. Yamamoto H, Tsubakihara Y. Limiting iron supplementation for anemia in dialysis patients—the Basis for Japan's conservative guidelines. Semin Dial. 2011;24(3):269–71.

12. Bohlius J, Bohlke K, Castelli R, et al. Management of cancer-associated anemia with erythropoiesis-stimulating agents: ASCO/ASH clinical practice guideline update. J Clin Oncol. 2019;37(15):1336–51.

13. KDIGO Clinical Practice Guideline Working Group. KDIGO clinical practice guideline for anemia in chronic kidney disease. Kidney Int. 2012;2:1–335.

14. Barratt J, Sulowicz W, Schömig M, et al. Efficacy and cardiovascular safety of roxadustat in dialysis-dependent chronic kidney disease: pooled analysis of four phase 3 studies. Adv Ther. 2021;38(10):5345–60.

15. Beck J, Henschel C, Chou J, Lin A, del Balzo U. Evaluation of the carcinogenic potential of roxadustat (FG-4592), a small molecule inhibitor of hypoxia-inducible factor prolyl hydroxylase in CD-1 mice and sprague dawley rats. Int J Toxicol. 2017;36(6):427–39.

16. Seeley TW, Sternlicht MD, Klaus SJ, Neff TB, Liu DY. Induction of erythropoiesis by hypoxia-inducible factor prolyl hydroxylase inhibitors without promotion of tumor initiation, progression, or metastasis in a VEGF-sensitive model of spontaneous breast cancer. Hypoxia (Auckland, NZ). 2017;5:1–9.

17. Glaspy J, Gabrail NY, Locantore-Ford P, et al. Open-label, Phase 2 study of roxadustat for the treatment of anemia in patients receiving chemotherapy for non-myeloid malignancies. Am J Hematol. 2023;98(5):703–11.

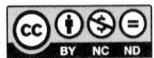

Treatment of Severe Anemia in an MPO-ANCA and Anti-GBM Double-Seropositive Patient

Wei-Wei Zhang, Jie Liu, Yan-Yun Xie, Qiong-Jing Yuan, and Xiang-Cheng Xiao

25.1 Case Presentation

A 56-year-old female patient was admitted to the Department of Nephrology because of acute kidney injury on December 16, 2022. Three months earlier, this patient went to the local hospital with a chief complaint of transient recurring generalized joint pain, but no abnormalities were found on routine blood examination (RBC $4.18 \times 10^{12}/L$, hemoglobin 121 g/L) or liver and renal function tests (albumin 46.4 g/L, creatinine 48.5 μmol/L); thus, no special treatments were administered. One month later, joint pain improved spontaneously, but she gradually experienced symptoms of abdominal distension and poor appetite, which were occasionally accompanied by vomiting after eating, low daily water intake, and a significantly reduced urine volume of approximately 50–100 ml per day, resulting in a dark urine color. The symptoms of systemic fatigue, abdominal distension, and poor appetite gradually worsened. On November 22, she was readmitted to the local hospital. Chronic cholecystitis with gallstones was showed by abdominal ultrasound, then given symptomatic treatment with omeprazole, but the symptoms of abdominal distension did not significantly improve. On December 7, 2022, she underwent gastroscopy examination and tissue biopsy at the local hospital, and the results showed a neuroendocrine tumor (stage G1) (gastric body). The patient then came to our hospital for further diagnosis and treatment, where outpatient examinations revealed a hemoglobin concentration of 73 g/L and a serum creatinine concentration of 1284.6 μmol/L. Hemodialysis therapy was started, and she was admitted to our nephrology department with acute kidney injury.

She had a history of chronic bronchitis for 20 years with no special treatment. No other special information on personal or family history was found. Her blood pressure was 130/72 mmHg, and her body weight was 56 kg. The physical examination

W.-W. Zhang · J. Liu · Y.-Y. Xie · Q.-J. Yuan (✉) · X.-C. Xiao (✉)
Department of Nephrology, Xiangya Hospital of Central South University, Changsha, China
e-mail: yuanqiongjing@csu.edu.cn; xiaoxc@csu.edu.cn

B.-C. Liu (ed.), *Treatment of Refractory Renal Anemia*,
https://doi.org/10.1007/978-981-97-7636-8_25

showed an anemic appearance with pale skin and mucous membranes. Auscultation revealed a weakened breath sound in both lungs and moist rales heard at the bottom of both lungs. There was mild edema in the face and both legs but no acropachy. Other physical examinations were normal.

The relevant detailed examinations were completed during hospitalization. Laboratory examinations revealed the following: nucleic acid detection of SARS-CoV-2 (+), WBC 5.7×10^9/L, RBC 1.97×10^9/L, hemoglobin 57.0 g/L, platelets 103×10^9/mL, granulocytes 1.58%, stool occult blood test (−), urinary occult blood (+++), urinary protein (+++), 24 h urine volume 0.2 L, 24 h total urinary protein 1.09 g, total serum protein 53.5 g/L, serum albumin 27.9 g/L, serum urea nitrogen 18.99 mmol/L, serum creatinine 916 μmol/L, ESR 42 mm/h, C-reactive protein 65.7 mg/L, calcitonin 0.35 ng/mL, parathyroid hormone 138.5 pg/mL, plasma fibrin degradation products 22.4 mg/L, D-dimer 2.08 mg/L, vitamin B12 325 pg/mL, folic acid 9.37 ng/mL, erythropoietin 81.65 mIU/mL, ferritin 228.8 ng/mL, serum iron 4.2 μmol/L, total iron-binding capacity 26 μmol/L, transferrin 1.13 g/L, and transferrin saturation 16.15%. Viral infections (hepatitis B and C or HIV infections), other autoantibodies (including anti-nuclear, anti-double-stranded DNA, etc.), blood and urine immunofixation by electrophoresis, and light chain determination were negative or normal. The electrocardiogram showed low T-waves. A pulmonary computed tomography (CT) scan showed bilateral diffuse infiltration, left pulmonary atelectasis, bilateral pleural effusion, bilateral bronchiectasis, and inflammation, with partial intraluminal sputum formation. Ultrasonography of the urinary system revealed kidney parenchymal lesions (grade A) and abdominal effusion. Ultrasonography of the heart showed an enlarged left atrium, a widened ascending aorta, thickening of the left ventricular wall, and aortic and mitral valve calcification with mild regurgitation. Gastric histopathological examination was performed again, and the results revealed a neuroendocrine tumor (stage G1) (fundus of the stomach). Based on the patient's medical history and the abovementioned examination results, the final diagnosis was MPO-ANCA and anti-GBM double-seropositive systemic vasculitis, rapidly progressive glomerulonephritis, bronchiectasis with infection, COVID-19, gastric neuroendocrine tumor (stage G1), chronic bronchitis, and gallstones with cholecystitis.

Treatment regimens included intensive hemodialysis with intermittent plasmapheresis (12 times), nirmatrelvir/ritonavir for COVID-19, and methylprednisolone (20 mg Qd ivgtt) to reduce inflammation. The patient had severe pulmonary lesions on admission, suggesting systemic vasculitis involving the lungs with severe infection. We strengthened antibacterial infection treatment based on anti-COVID-19 therapy, but pulmonary CT showed more pulmonary lesions and bilateral pleural effusion than before, and viral pneumonia still occurred. The symptoms of cough and hemoptysis during hospitalization were aggravated, and sputum culture results showed Gram-negative bacilli and fungal infections in the respiratory tract. Pulmonary CT after combined antifungal treatment showed that the grinding-glass shadow range of both lungs had decreased, but the consolidation range had increased. Vasculitis advanced rapidly and continuously aggravated renal and lung damage in this patient. Therefore, after controlling the patient's infection symptoms, immunosuppressive treatment was given immediately, while hemodialysis and intermittent plasma exchange therapy were continued. This patient received a cyclophosphamide immunosuppressive regimen, which was administered monthly over 4 months with a cumulative dose of 2.2 g (cyclophosphamide 0.4 g in January 2023, 0.6 g in February 2023, 0.4 g in March 2023, and 0.8 g in April 2023). The patient was admitted with severe anemia (57 g/L). Renal anemia is the predominant type of anti-neutrophil cytoplasmic antibody (ANCA)-associated renal vasculitis. Therefore, the patient was treated with a large dose of erythropoietin (1 wu qw) supplemented with an intermittent infusion of concentrated red blood cells. The patient had abnormal iron metabolism, but iron was not supplemented during the acute phase of infection. One month after erythropoiesis-stimulating agent (ESA) treatment, anemia did not improve, and hemoglobin fluctuated at 57–67 g/L in this patient. The re-examination of the anti-MPO antibody was 37.48 IU/mL; the anti-GBM antibody was 42.19 IU/mL, and pulmonary CT re-examination was basically the same as before. ESAs had a weak effect against anemia in this patient. Based on guidelines and clinical experience, the treatment of anemia was switched to the HIF-PHI drug roxadustat on 13 January 2023, with a standard dose of 100 mg three times weekly. During the follow-up period, the hemoglobin level increased steadily and reached 134 g/L after 3 months of roxadustat treatment, so the dose was reduced to 50 mg three times weekly. In addition, the condition of the lungs of the patient significantly improved, and CT re-examination showed that the grinding-glass shadow and consolidation range of both lungs were significantly reduced. Surprisingly, the anti-GBM antibody level also decreased to the normal range as her anemia improved. The patient's hemoglobin is now stable at approximately 120 g/L (Fig. 25.1).

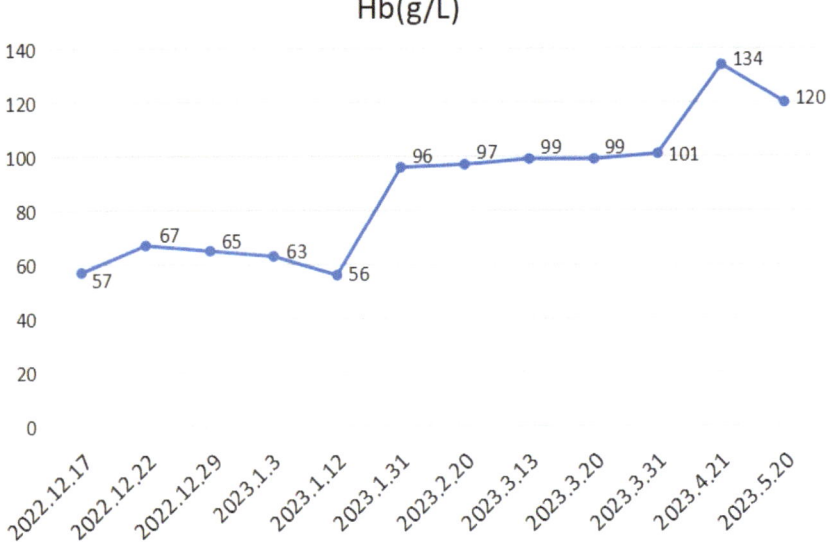

Fig. 25.1   Changes in hemoglobin levels

25.2 Discussion

This is a middle-aged female patient with MPO-ANCA and anti-GBM double-seropositive ANCA-associated vasculitis (AAV). Compared with isolated MPO-ANCAs or anti-GBM-positive patients, patients with double-positive AAVs have faster progression and worse renal outcomes due to renal damage, as well as severe and wider organ involvement [1, 2]. In this patient, kidney and lung involvement was severe, and kidney damage manifested as rapidly progressive nephritic syndrome. Inflammation of small vessels in the lungs constantly invaded the lung tissue, and complex pulmonary infections hindered the use of immunosuppressants. Anemia is a common complication of AAV and is an important factor affecting the prognosis of AAV patients [3]. During hospitalization, high-dose ESA and intermittent blood transfusion treatments had no significant effect on our patient's anemia or autoantibody levels. She was switched to oral roxadustat for anemia and then received monthly cyclophosphamide immunosuppression therapy, and her Hb level increased steadily and is currently at a normal level. Therefore, this case study demonstrates that roxadustat is beneficial for the treatment of immune-inflammatory disease-related anemia.

Anemia has been reported as a complication of autoimmune and inflammatory diseases. Anemia that occurs in the context of autoimmune and inflammatory diseases is known as anemia of chronic disease (ACD). The mechanisms of ACD include changes in iron metabolism, inadequate erythropoiesis, and shortening of the erythrocyte lifespan. Complications associated with ACD include infections, malignancies, autoimmune diseases, chronic rejection after transplantation, and chronic kidney disease (CKD) [4]. ACD is an important complication of ANCA-associated renal vasculitis, and the causes of anemia in patients with ANCA-associated renal vasculitis are expected to be multifactorial. Anemia has already been described in most patients with ANCA-associated renal vasculitis, renal anemia being the predominant type. The combination of severe anemia and ANCA-associated renal vasculitis has been shown to lead to poor long-term renal prognosis and a shortened lifespan [3, 5]. MPO-AAV in anti-GBM seropositive individuals mainly affects older people and usually causes multiorgan injury. Bowman's capsule rupture is seen more frequently in such patients. Renal and survival outcomes are worse in serological double-seropositive patients than in MPO-AAV patients. Therefore, MPO-ANCA-/anti-GBM-double-seropositive patients have much fewer normal glomeruli than MPO-AAV-single-positive patients, making them more prone to severe renal anemia and aggravating the progression of the disease [1, 6].

The 2012 Kidney Disease: Improving Global Outcomes (KDIGO) guidelines recommend ESAs as the primary treatment for renal anemia, but with the emergence of evidence of ESA-related adverse outcomes, ESAs have become gradually less used, while iron supplementation has become more common in clinical practice for treating renal anemia in recent years [7, 8]. In this MPO-ANCA-/anti-GBM-double-seropositive patient, MPO-ANCA and anti-GBM antibody caused a double hit on the glomerular vessels and basement membrane, significantly decreasing the normal glomerular ratio and causing rapid progression to end-stage renal disease (ESRD). Consequently, this patient had extremely high serum creatinine combined with severe anemia at first admission. Moreover, severe persistent pulmonary infections and the use of immunosuppressants aggravate ACD complicated by AAV, which in turn aggravates infections, immune-inflammatory disorders, and the progression of CKD, forming a vicious cycle and significantly reducing the therapeutic responsiveness to ESAs. In addition, thrombotic events are very common in AAV, mainly due to vascular endothelial damage caused by inflammatory factors, blood hypercoagulability induced by complement activation, and concomitant elevation of antiphospholipid antibodies. AAV patients are at extremely high risk of arteriovenous thrombosis [9, 10]. However, the long-term use of ESAs can promote thromboembolism and even increase the risk of cardiovascular events and death [11, 12]. Compared with the general population, patients with AAV have an increased risk of malignancy, especially patients receiving immunosuppressive treatment regimens with cyclophosphamide [13]. This patient not only received regular immunosuppressive therapy with cyclophosphamide but also had a precancerous lesion and a gastric neuroendocrine tumor in the G1 stage with a high risk of malignancy. However, long-term use of ESAs may also promote tumor malignancy [11]. In summary, the long-term use of ESAs is not suitable for the treatment of AAV-related renal anemia in this patient.

Hypoxia-inducible factor prolyl hydroxylase inhibitors (HIF-PHIs), a new generation of drugs for renal anemia with novel mechanisms, can induce erythropoiesis by stimulating the production of endogenous erythropoietin and promoting iron utilization through HIF, which also has potential benefits, including hypolipidemic, antihypertensive, and anti-inflammatory effects, preventing ischemic injury, and delaying the progression of CKD. Compared to ESAs, they have an efficacy and dose requirements that are less affected by the inflammatory state of the body, and phase II and III clinical trials have shown that they are comparable to ESAs in terms of anemia correction and maintenance, with better safety profiles for cardiovascular events, thrombosis, malignancy, and mortality [14–16]. Currently, five HIF-PHIs, namely, roxadustat, daprodustat, vadadustat, molidustat, and enarodustat, have been approved in China and Japan for the treatment of anemia in patients with CKD, with roxadustat being the most effective at increasing hemoglobin and lowering ferritin levels [17]. According to the KDIGO guidelines [18] and the Asia Pacific Society of Nephrology (APSN) [19], as an alternative to ESAs, HIF-PHIs can be applied to correct and maintain hemoglobin levels in patients with renal anemia. Therefore, shortly after the initiation of cyclophosphamide immunosuppressive therapy, we switched our patient to roxadustat for continued treatment of anemia, and over 3 months of treatment at standard doses, the patient's hemoglobin level increased steadily to 134 g/L. Since high hemoglobin may promote thrombosis in patients with vasculitis, such as ours, we reduced the roxadustat dose. Despite the patient's long-term immunosuppressive therapy and recurrent pulmonary infections, the treatment of anemia with roxadustat was not effective. Additionally, with the improvement of anemia, the patient's primary autoimmune disease was alleviated to some extent, manifested in the remission of hematuria and hemoptysis, a decrease in the serum MPO-ANCA and anti-GBM levels, and a reduction in the number of lung lesions. Currently, the patient's hemoglobin is within the normal range, with no cardiovascular events, thrombosis, or malignancy during follow-up.

Roxadustat has gained increasing prominence in the treatment of anemia in CKD patients, and extensive clinical experience has been accumulated. However, there is too little clinical evidence to support the effectiveness and safety of roxadustat in patients with renal disease complicated by various refractory and ESA-resistant anemias. To establish optimal anemia management strategies for HIF-PHIs, a variety of aspects, including long-term safety, appropriate hemoglobin level targets, and which types of patients will benefit from these new drugs, need to be evaluated in future studies.

In this MPO-ANCA-/anti-GBM-double-seropositive vasculitis patient with severe kidney injury, immunoinflammatory disorders, and severe infections, immunosuppressive agents aggravated her anemia and decreased her responsiveness to ESAs. Roxadustat is less affected by the inflammatory state of the body and thus can treat renal anemia in patients with ANCA-associated renal vasculitis safely and effectively, which provides valuable experience in the treatment of anemia in patients with immune kidney diseases.

References

1. Srivastava A, Rao GK, Segal PE, et al. Characteristics and outcome of crescentic glomerulonephritis in patients with both antineutrophil cytoplasmic antibody and anti-glomerular basement membrane antibody. Clin Rheumatol. 2013;32(9):1317–22.
2. Geetha D, Jefferson JA. ANCA-associated vasculitis: core curriculum 2020. Am J Kidney Dis. 2020;75(1):124–37.
3. Kawamura T, Usui J, Kaneko S, et al. Anaemia is an essential complication of ANCA-associated renal vasculitis: a single center cohort study. BMC Nephrol. 2017;18(1):337.
4. Weiss G, Goodnough LT. Anemia of chronic disease. N Engl J Med. 2005;352(10):1011–23.
5. Baier E, Tampe D, Hakroush S, et al. Low levels of hemoglobin associate with critical illness and predict disease course in patients with ANCA-associated renal vasculitis. Sci Rep. 2022;12(1):18736.
6. Hu X, Shen C, Meng T, et al. Clinical features and prognosis of MPO-ANCA and anti-GBM double-seropositive patients. Front Immunol. 2022;13:991469.
7. Babitt JL, Eisenga MF, Haase VH, et al. Controversies in optimal anemia management: conclusions from a kidney disease: improving global outcomes (KDIGO) conference. Kidney Int. 2021;99(6):1280–95.
8. Thavarajah S, Choi MJ. The use of erythropoiesis-stimulating agents in patients with CKD and cancer: a clinical approach. Am J Kidney Dis. 2019;74(5):667–74.
9. Misra DP, Thomas KN, Gasparyan AY, et al. Mechanisms of thrombosis in ANCA-associated vasculitis. Clin Rheumatol. 2021;40(12):4807–15.
10. Huang YM, Wang H, Wang C, et al. Promotion of hypercoagulability in antineutrophil cytoplasmic antibody-associated vasculitis by C5a-induced tissue factor-expressing microparticles and neutrophil extracellular traps. Arthritis Rheumatol. 2015;67(10):2780–90.
11. Barbera L, Thomas G. Erythropoiesis stimulating agents, thrombosis and cancer. Radiother Oncol. 2010;95(3):269–76.
12. Drüeke TB, Massy ZA. Erythropoiesis-stimulating agents and mortality. J Am Soc Nephrol. 2019;30(6):907–8.
13. Trejo MACW, Bajema IM, van Daalen EE. Antineutrophil cytoplasmic antibody-associated vasculitis and malignancy. Curr Opin Rheumatol. 2018;30(1):44–9.
14. Sugahara M, Tanaka T, Nangaku M. Future perspectives of anemia management in chronic kidney disease using hypoxia-inducible factor-prolyl hydroxylase inhibitors. Pharmacol Ther. 2022;239:108272.

15. Mima A. Hypoxia-inducible factor-prolyl hydroxylase inhibitors for renal anemia in chronic kidney disease: advantages and disadvantages. Eur J Pharmacol. 2021;912:174583.
16. Locatelli F, Del Vecchio L. Hypoxia-inducible factor-prolyl hydroxyl domain inhibitors: from theoretical superiority to clinical noninferiority compared with current ESAs? J Am Soc Nephrol. 2022;33(11):1966–79.
17. Chen J, Shou X, Xu Y, et al. A network meta-analysis of the efficacy of hypoxia-inducible factor prolyl-hydroxylase inhibitors in dialysis chronic kidney disease. Aging. 2023;15(6):2237–74.
18. Ku E, Del Vecchio L, Eckardt KU, et al. Novel anemia therapies in chronic kidney disease: conclusions from a kidney disease: improving global outcomes (KDIGO) controversies conference. Kidney Int. 2023;104(4):655–80.
19. Yap DYH, McMahon LP, Hao CM, et al. Recommendations by the Asian Pacific society of nephrology (APSN) on the appropriate use of HIF-PH inhibitors. Nephrology (Carlton). 2021;26(2):105–18.

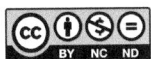

Is Roxadustat Responsible for the Jaundice of a Dialysis Patient with β-Thalassemia? A Case Report

26

Hong-Shan Zhou, Han-Wei Huang, Hui Xu, Gong Xiao, and Qiong-Jing Yuan

26.1 Case Presentation

A 54-year-old woman was admitted with anemia and fatigue for more than 10 years in January 2018. The patient had a history of hypertension and chronic kidney disease (CKD) secondary to chronic glomerulonephritis for 4 years. She regularly took antihypertensive drugs and began continuous ambulatory peritoneal dialysis in 2016.

Laboratory examinations showed a white blood cell (WBC) count of $2.4 \times 10^9/L$, red blood cell (RBC) count of $2.07 \times 10^9/L$, platelet (PLT) count of $89 \times 10^9/L$, hemoglobin (Hb) concentration of 43g/L, mean corpuscular volume (MCV) of 67.9 fl, mean corpuscular hemoglobin (MCH) of 20.8 PG, and mean corpuscular hemoglobin concentration (MCHC) of 306.6 g/L. Analysis of iron metabolism showed that her serum iron was 10.7 μmol/L, transferrin 0.84 g/L, serum total iron-binding capacity 20.8 μmol/L, and ferritin 1661 μg/L. Bone marrow aspiration showed bone marrow hyperplasia, high erythrocytes, and low granulocytes and platelets. She was diagnosed with renal anemia and stage 5 CKD. As a result, she was treated with 3000 u erythropoietin (EPO) once a week and 0.15 g polysaccharide iron complex once a day for anemia since January 2017. Despite one year of treatment, she still presented with anemia, and her hemoglobin did not increase beyond 70 g/L, even after multiple blood transfusions and increasing the dose of EPO to 10,000 u twice weekly.

The patient was readmitted with severe anemia with fatigue and bilateral lower extremity edema in December 2021. Laboratory examinations revealed a WBC of $1.9 \times 10^9/L$, RBC of $2.28 \times 10^9/L$, PLT of $44 \times 10^9/L$, and Hb of 49g/L. Bone marrow aspiration and biopsy were recommended for anemia, but she refused, and treatment was switched to 120 mg of roxadustat thrice weekly based on her weight

H.-S. Zhou · H.-W. Huang · H. Xu (✉) · G. Xiao · Q.-J. Yuan (✉)
Department of Nephrology, Xiangya Hospital of Central South University, Changsha, Hunan, China
e-mail: xuhuiye@csu.edu.cn; yuanqiongjing@csu.edu.cn

© The Author(s) 2025
B.-C. Liu (ed.), *Treatment of Refractory Renal Anemia*,
https://doi.org/10.1007/978-981-97-7636-8_26

of 62.5 kg. Her hemoglobin increased to 89 g/L after one week. After 8 months of treatment with roxadustat, she returned to the hospital with her hemoglobin level reaching 151 g/L.

However, in August 2022, the patient presented with jaundice without a belly-ache, bleeding, or infection. Her blood pressure was 90/50 mmHg. The physical examination suggested yellow skin, mucosa, and sclera. The complete blood counts were as follows: WBC count of 4.2×10^9/L, RBC count of 5.95×10^9/L, PLT count of 57×10^9/L, and Hb concentration of 133 g/L. Her hepatic function indices were as follows: total bilirubin (TB) 380 µmol/L, conjugated bilirubin (CB) 239.4 µmol/L, total bile acid 17.5 µmol/L, alanine aminotransferase (ALT) 91.9 U/L, and aspartate aminotransferase (AST) 174.8 U/L. Immune-associated antibodies, including anti-nuclear Ab, anti-neutrophilic cytoplasmic Ab, and anticardiolipin Ab, were nega-tive. Hepatitis B and hepatitis C serology results were also negative. No abnormalities in the levels of tumor markers, such as α-fetoprotein (AFP) or carcinoembryonic antigen (CEA), were detected. Further imaging revealed no signs of space-occupying lesions in the liver or extrahepatic vessels. The ratio of CB to TB was 0.63, which indicated obstructive jaundice. Based on the test results, the patient was diagnosed with obstructive jaundice due to the possibility of intrahepatic vascular microthrombosis.

Genetic testing suggested heterozygous β-thalassemia. No chromosomal anoma-lies were found in the bone marrow. The patient was diagnosed with thalassemia. Roxadustat was discontinued, and the treatment for anemia was then switched to intermittent blood transfusions. Moreover, she underwent plasmapheresis. After one week of symptomatic treatment and plasmapheresis, bilirubin decreased to 309.4 µmol/L. After 3 weeks of treatment, the jaundice had significantly improved; her Hb level was 78 g/L, and her bilirubin had returned to 249.7 µmol/L. One month after follow-up, the total bilirubin level had returned to the normal range.

26.2 Discussion

A middle-aged female was repeatedly admitted due to severe anemia and a history of CKD and hypertension. To correct her anemia, a high dose of EPO and blood transfusions were given, which she responded poorly either. Thus, roxadustat was prescribed as an alternative treatment. However, there was failure to promptly adjust medication dosage due to irregular follow-up appointments despite a 20 kg weight loss of the patient. The hemoglobin level reached 151 g/L. Unfortunately, she expe-rienced jaundice after her hemoglobin level increased to normal. To explore the cause of her jaundice, she underwent genetic testing, which suggested β-thalassemia，so she switched to receive intermittent blood transfusions.

In China, the prevalence of β-thalassemia is approximately 1–6% [1], but the prevalence of β-thalassemia in CKD patients is not well known. As an autosomal recessive disease, β-thalassemia is associated with low or absent β-globin chain synthesis [2], which leads to hemolysis and ineffective erythropoiesis [3]. β-Thalassemia is categorized into β-thalassemia major (BTM), β-thalassemia intermedia (BTI), or β-thalassemia minor (carriers) [4]. BTI patients may be asymptomatic until adulthood, and anemia is milder in these patients than in BTM patients, which means that they have no or only occasional blood transfusions in their early years [2, 5]. The cornerstones of treatments for β-thalassemia are blood transfusion and iron chelation therapy (ICT), which can improve life expectancy [4].

Erythropoiesis-stimulating agents (ESAs) have been widely used for treating renal anemia, and a considerable proportion of ESA-hyporesponsive patients keep taking these agents. The known causes of ESA hyporesponsiveness include infection, a chronic inflammatory state, iron deficiency, etc. Importantly, hemoglobinopathies are involved [6]. Roxadustat is a novel anti-anemia drug that acts through multiple pathways. As a hypoxia-inducible factor (HIF) prolyl hydroxylase inhibitor aimed at increasing HIF activity, roxadustat upregulates proteins such as erythropoietin, erythropoietin receptor, enzymes involved in heme biosynthesis, and iron absorption- and transport-related proteins, which coordinately promote erythropoiesis [7]. Two large cohort studies in China demonstrated that roxadustat was effective in correcting anemia in CKD patients who did or did not undergo dialysis [7, 8]. A clinical trial also revealed that roxadustat had potential benefits on patients with ESA-induced hyporesponsive CKD [9]. For patients with CKD complicated with thalassemia and poor response to EPO, two cases reported that roxadustat can effectively increase hemoglobin [10, 11]. A prospective, randomized controlled study in China targeting similar patients also showed that roxadustat improved anemia better than EPO and effectively increased iron utilization by promoting the production of endogenous EPO, regulating ferritin levels, and suppressing the inflammatory response [12].

Notably, β-thalassemia is a hereditary anemia caused by genetic mutations. Its abnormal hemoglobin structure results in chronic hemolysis, a condition that current drugs cannot cure. Even with increased erythropoiesis, the production of globin chains may remain imbalanced. Besides, elevated hemoglobin levels more than 150 g/L significantly elevate the risk of adverse events for patients, including hypertension and thrombosis events [13]. More clinical evidence are needed to determine the side effect of roxadustat on patient with β-thalassemia. Thalassemia can have many complications. The high prevalence of thromboembolic events due to hypercoagulable state in BTI is gaining attention [14]. Abnormal red blood cells contribute to a hypercoagulable state [14]. Bilirubin, mainly conjugated bilirubin, was elevated in the current patient. Therefore, in addition to hemolysis, we speculated that intrahepatic vascular microthrombosis caused by increased abnormal RBCs leads to obstructive jaundice.

In summary, the anemia of the patient aggravated by BTI and CKD may be the reason she responded strongly to roxadustat. Therefore, the accompanying severe hemolysis and the possible process of microvascular thrombosis led to jaundice in this patient. The cause of anemia in CKD patients can coexist, not simply renal anemia, such as β-thalassemia in this case. For similar patients, roxadustat may exacerbate hemolysis, which means more cautious prescriptions. On the other hand, when anemia patients experience hemolysis after using roxadustat, we must also consider the possibility of hemoglobinopathies.

References

1. Xu X, Wu X. Epidemiology and treatment of beta thalassemia major in China. Pediatr Investig. 2019;4(1):43–7.
2. Origa R. β-thalassemia. Genet Med. 2017;19(6):609–19.
3. Weatherall DJ. Phenotype—genotype relationships in monogenic disease: lessons from the thalassaemias. Nat Rev Genet. 2001;2(4):245–55.
4. Shah FT, Sayani F, Trompeter S, Drasar E, Piga A. Challenges of blood transfusions in β-thalassemia. Blood Rev. 2019;37:100588.
5. Cappellini MD, Cohen A, Porter J, Taher A, Viprakasit V. Guidelines for the management of Transfusion Dependent Thalassaemia (TDT). Nicosia, CY: Thalassaemia International Federation; 2014.
6. Macdougall IC, Cooper AC. Erythropoietin resistance: the role of inflammation and pro-inflammatory cytokines. Nephrol Dial Transplant. 2002;17(suppl_11):39–43.
7. Chen N, Hao C, Peng X, et al. Roxadustat for anemia in patients with kidney disease not receiving dialysis. N Engl J Med. 2019;381(11):1001–10.
8. Chen N, Hao C, Liu BC, et al. Roxadustat treatment for anemia in patients undergoing long-term dialysis. N Engl J Med. 2019;381(11):1011–22.
9. Akizawa T, Tanaka-Amino K, Otsuka T, Yamaguchi Y. Factors affecting doses of roxadustat versus darbepoetin alfa for anemia in nondialysis patients. Am J Nephrol. 2021;52(9):702–13.
10. Liu Y, LI NY, Zhang Q, et al. Hypoxia-inducible factor prolyl hydroxylase inhibitor in the treatment of thalassemia with renal anemia: a case report. Fudan Univ J Med Sci. 2022,49(01):156–58.
11. Wang KM, Chen J. Effective use of Roxadustat in the treatment of β-thalassemia with renal anemia: a case report. Pract J of Clin Med. 2022,19(06):214–15.
12. Zhou HY, Zhou Y, Wang YY, et al. Effect of Roxadustat on anemia and iron metabolism in patients with chronic kidney disease complicated with thalassemia. Chin J Pract Intern Med. 2023,43(11):915–27.
13. Chen H, Cheng Q, Wang J, Zhao X, Zhu S. Long-term efficacy and safety of hypoxia-inducible factor prolyl hydroxylase inhibitors in anaemia of chronic kidney disease: a meta-analysis including 13,146 patients. J Clin Pharm Ther. 2021;46(4):999–1009.
14. Taher AT, Otrock ZK, Uthman I, Cappellini MD. Thalassemia and hypercoagulability. Blood Rev. 2008;22(5):283–92.

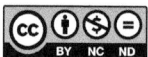

Treatment of Anemia in a Patient with Chronic Kidney Disease and Cerebral Infarction

27

Wen Zheng, Dong-Wei Liu, and Zhang-Suo Liu

27.1 Case Presentation

A 29-year-old man had elevated serum creatinine because of sudden cerebral infarction 3 months before admission. Serum creatinine was 336.8 μmol/L, and he was started on drugs to improve circulation and to protect the kidney. Two weeks earlier, he complained of poor appetite and fatigue and presented to the local hospital. Laboratory tests revealed serum creatinine 400 μmol/L, hemoglobin 105 g/L, and albumin 45.5 g/L. For further treatment, the patient was referred to our hospital.

He had a history of hypertension for more than 5 years with a maximum blood pressure of 200/100 mmHg, and his blood pressure was kept between 140–150/90–100 mmHg under five oral antihypertensive drugs. He also had a history of cerebral infarction 3 months earlier, regularly took aspirin and atorvastatin, and had difficulty moving his left limbs. His body weight was 110 kg, his height was 172 cm, and his body mass index (BMI) was 37.1 kg/m^2.

After admission, his laboratory findings revealed WBC 6.52×10^9/L, RBC 3.25×10^{12}/L, hemoglobin 95 g/L, platelets 214×10^9/L, blood urea nitrogen 19.99 mmol/L, serum creatinine 351 μmol/L (normal, 20–115 μmol/L), uric acid 456 μmol/L, serum calcium 2.34 mmol/L, phosphorus 2.13 mmol/L, total protein 66.5 g/L, and albumin 41.5 g/L. A morning urinalysis revealed 2+ protein, and the protein level in 24-h urine was 0.86 g. C-reactive protein was 0.8 mg/L, and PTH was 74.1 pg/mL. Serologic indicators, such as autoantibodies (including anti-nuclear, anti-double-stranded DNA, anti-GBM, and anti-neutrophil

W. Zheng · D.-W. Liu (✉) · Z.-S. Liu (✉)
Department of Integrated Traditional and Western Nephrology, The First Affiliated Hospital of Zhengzhou University, Zhengzhou, People's Republic of China
e-mail: liu-dongwei@zzu.edu.cn

© The Author(s) 2025
B.-C. Liu (ed.), *Treatment of Refractory Renal Anemia*,
https://doi.org/10.1007/978-981-97-7636-8_27

167

cytoplasmic antibodies), anti-phospholipase A2 receptor, and tumor markers, were all negative. There were no obvious abnormalities in the results of urine protein electrophoresis or serum protein electrophoresis. Ultrasound showed bilateral diffuse renal echo changes (right kidney, 9.6 cm in length; left kidney, 9.5 cm in length).

To clarify the pathological changes in his kidney histology, a renal biopsy was performed. Combined with light microscopic examination, immunofluorescence, and electron microscopy, the results revealed obesity-related focal segmental glomerulosclerosis as the primary diagnosis and malignant hypertensive renal damage as the secondary diagnosis. For treatment, drugs for hypotension, anticoagulation, and circulation improvement were administered.

In addition, the patient had mild anemia with a hemoglobin of 95 g/L. Iron status biomarkers were detected, and there was no obvious iron deficiency (iron 9.53 μmol/L, total iron-binding capacity 39.53 μmol/L, and transferrin saturation (TSAT) 24%). Considering the patient's past medical history and clinical laboratory results, we prescribed a standard dosage of roxadustat (100 mg for ≥60 kg) thrice a week. After the initial treatment, the hemoglobin increased gradually to 124 g/L. Then, we adjusted the dose of roxadustat to 70 mg thrice a week according to the instructions. During the 8-month follow-up, the patient's hemoglobin decreased to 110 g/L and stayed at 110–116 g/L. However, the hemoglobin decreased to 90 g/L because the patient reduced the dose of roxadustat to 50 mg thrice a week. Moreover, the patient had absolute iron deficiency (iron 4.62 μmol/L, total iron-binding capacity 64.82 μmol/L, and TAST 7%). Thus, iron supplementation and 100 mg roxadustat thrice a week were given to correct his anemia. The changes in hemoglobin are shown in Fig. 27.1. The changes in body weight, serum creatinine level, and indicators of ferric metabolism are shown in Table 27.1.

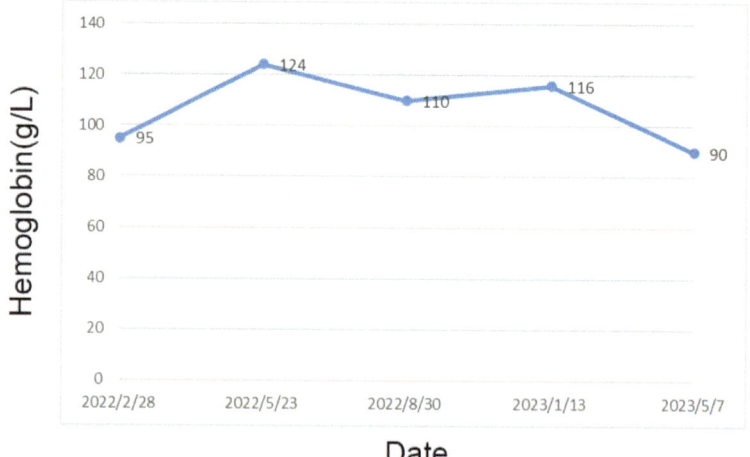

Fig. 27.1 The changes in hemoglobin levels

Table 27.1 Changes in body weight, serum creatinine level, and indicators of ferric metabolism

	Body weight(kg)	Scr (μmol/L)	Iron (μmol/L)	Ferritin (μg/L)	TIBC (μmol/L)	TSAT (%)
2022-02-28	110	351	9.53	243.3	39.53	24
2022-05-23	98	300	9.56	244.4	50.66	18.8
2022-08-30	95	292	–	–	–	–
2023-01-13	88	257	–	–	–	–
2023-05-07	88	295	4.62	15.3	64.82	7

27.2 Discussion

Renal anemia is a common complication of CKD, especially ESRD, and is predominantly caused by a reduced EPO production by the kidney. Renal anemia can occur at any stage of CKD, but its prevalence and severity increase with the progression of CKD [1]. This is a young male patient with stage 4 CKD who presented with mild anemia and a history of cerebral infarction and malignant hypertension. Renal biopsy showed obesity-related focal segmental glomerulosclerosis at the primary diagnosis and malignant hypertensive renal damage at the secondary diagnosis. To avoid negative effects on blood pressure and cerebrovascular risk, the patient was given roxadustat instead of an ESA to correct his anemia. At the beginning of treatment, there was no obvious iron deficiency, and only roxadustat was prescribed. The patient responded well, and his hemoglobin gradually increased to the target level.

ESAs have been widely used to maintain optimal hemoglobin levels in patients with both dialysis and nondialysis CKD [2]. They can also delay the progression of chronic kidney disease, reduce hospitalization and all-cause mortality, and improve the quality of life of CKD patients. However, ESAs also have adverse effects. For example, ESAs can increase blood pressure. High-dose ESAs can increase the risks of cardiovascular events and infection, as well as hospitalizations and mortality. Compared with rHuEPO, roxadustat had less influence on blood pressure in peritoneal dialysis patients with renal anemia [3]. In addition, ESA resistance can occur in some patients, resulting in treatment failure. According to the TREAT study [4], the use of ESAs should be avoided in patients with a history of stroke, as both history of stroke and ESA treatment are independent risk factors for new stroke. Our patient had a history of cerebral infarction 3 months earlier, so roxadustat was chosen to correct his anemia.

Roxadustat is a novel oral hypoxia-inducible factor (HIF) prolyl hydroxylase inhibitor that increases endogenous erythropoietin concentrations by stabilizing HIF, and it has been recently endorsed for the treatment of anemia in CKD patients [5]. Recent randomized, multicenter, double-blind clinical studies done in China have shown that roxadustat significantly improved the hemoglobin level in CKD patients on and not on dialysis [6, 7]. Additionally, roxadustat was demonstrated to reduce serum cholesterol levels in a dose-dependent manner regardless of baseline statin use, which is beneficial for patients with metabolic syndrome [8]. The results of three randomized clinical trials showed that roxadustat treated continuously for ≥2 years was more effective than placebo in patients with anemia of nondialysis-dependent CKD [9]. Despite the proven short-term benefits of roxadustat in CKD patients, its long-term effect on clinical outcomes and socioeconomic burden needs further study.

Roxadustat is indicated to improve patient iron metabolism via multiple pathways. It increases iron absorption from the gastrointestinal tract, enhances the release of iron from hepatocytes, and increases the total serum binding capacity of iron [10]. A phase 3 clinical study reported that roxadustat reduced serum ferritin and TSAT in patients with nondialysis CKD [11]. However, a recent retrospective analysis found that ferritin levels and TSAT decreased at the early stage and increased in the late phase. In this case, the patient lost too much weight, resulting in nutritional deficiencies in the late phase. Thus, to increase the hemoglobin level, iron supplementation was given to correct the anemia.

Here, we report a renal anemia patient with a history of cerebral infarction and malignant hypertension, who was not suitable for the ESA treatment. In the initial treatment, oral roxadustat corrected anemia effectively and safely. However, an uncorrected reduction in roxadustat caused further aggravation of anemia, which may be corrected by increasing the dose of roxadustat and iron supplementation.

References

1. Go AS, Yang J, Ackerson LM, et al. Hemoglobin level, chronic kidney disease, and the risks of death and hospitalization in adults with chronic heart failure. Circulation. 2006;113(23):2713–23.
2. Raichoudhury R, Spinowitz BS. Treatment of anemia in difficult-to-manage patients with chronic kidney disease. Int J Geogr Inf Sci. 2021;11(1):26–34.
3. Cheng SQ, Zhou TT, Zhang ZH, et al. Roxadustat and recombinant human erythropoietin treatment on blood pressure and cardio-cerebrovascular complications in patients undergoing peritoneal dialysis. Chin J Nephrol Dial Transplant. 2022;31(1):9–14.
4. Skali H, Parving HH, Parfrey PS, et al. Stroke in patients with type 2 diabetes mellitus, chronic kidney disease, and anemia treated with Darbepoetin Alfa: the trial to reduce cardiovascular events with Aranesp therapy (TREAT) experience. Circulation. 2011;124(25):2903–8.
5. Chen D, Niu Y, Liu F, et al. Safety of HIF prolyl hydroxylase inhibitors for anemia in dialysis patients: a systematic review and network meta-analysis. Front Pharmacol. 2023;14:1163908.
6. Chen N, Hao C, Peng X, et al. Roxadustat for anemia in patients with kidney disease not receiving dialysis. N Engl J Med. 2019;381(11):1001–10.
7. Chen N, Hao C, Liu BC, et al. Roxadustat treatment for anemia in patients undergoing long-term dialysis. N Engl J Med. 2019;381(11):1011–22.
8. Takada A, Shibata T, Shiga T, et al. Pharmacokinetic/pharmacodynamic modeling of roxadustat's effect on LDL cholesterol in patients in Japan with dialysis-dependent chronic kidney disease and anemia. Drug Metab Pharmacokinet. 2022;46:100461.
9. Provenzano R, Szczech L, Leong R, et al. Efficacy and cardiovascular safety of roxadustat for treatment of anemia in patients with non-dialysis-dependent CKD: pooled results of three randomized clinical trials. Clin J Am Soc Nephrol. 2021;16(8):1190–200.
10. Gupta N, Wish JB. Hypoxia-inducible factor prolyl hydroxylase inhibitors: a potential new treatment for anemia in patients with CKD. Am J Kidney Dis. 2017;69(6):815–26.
11. Hirai K, Kaneko S, Minato S, et al. Effects of roxadustat on anemia, iron metabolism, and lipid metabolism in patients with non-dialysis chronic kidney disease. Front Med. 2023;10:1071342.

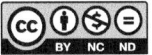

Roxadustat Corrects Acute Phosphate Nephropathy with Concurrent Renal Anemia: A Case Report

28

Xiao-Wan Liang, Li You, and Jun Xue

28.1 Case Presentation

A 61-year-old male patient with a history of hypertension and hyperuricemia was admitted with elevated serum creatinine on March 18, 2019. In January 2019, physical examination revealed a creatinine of 248 μmol/L, uric acid of 0.63 mmol/L, and hemoglobin of 86 g/L. There was no hematuria, foamy urine or decreased urine output, fever, nausea, low back pain, edema, or other symptoms and no further examination or treatment. In February 2019, the patient visited our outpatient clinic for follow-up, and reexamination showed a creatinine concentration of 220 μmol/L and a urinary microalbumin/creatinine ratio of 58.45 mg/g. On inquiry of his medical history, the patient had a creatinine level of 77 μmol/L during physical examination in May 2018. In November 2018, he underwent enteroscopy and oral sodium phosphate for bowel preparation. To further clarify the cause of the patient's abnormal renal function, no anemia-related treatment was administered before hospitalization.

The patient was in generally good health. He had a history of hypertension for more than 10 years, with his highest blood pressure being 160/90 mmHg. His blood pressure was well controlled by oral administration of amlodipine and angiotensin receptor blocker (ARB). After admission, the ARB was discontinued due to increased creatinine. He had elevated blood uric acid and oral benzbromarone without gout attacks. In January 2019, the patient had elevated blood lipids on physical examination and was treated with atorvastatin calcium lipid-lowering therapy. The patient had a *Helicobacter pylori* infection and was treated with a four-drug regimen in October 2018. The patient denied any history of infectious diseases, surgeries, blood transfusions, or allergies, except for quinolone antibiotics, and had no family history of genetic diseases. The physical examination findings were within

X.-W. Liang · L. You · J. Xue (✉)
Institute of Nephrology, Hua Shan Hospital, Fudan University, Shanghai, China
e-mail: xuejun@fudan.edu.cn

© The Author(s) 2025
B.-C. Liu (ed.), *Treatment of Refractory Renal Anemia*,
https://doi.org/10.1007/978-981-97-7636-8_28

normal limits, with no signs of anemia, edema, abnormal liver or spleen enlargement, or limb swelling, or normal muscle strength or tone.

Laboratory examinations revealed a white blood cell count of 5.71×10^9/L, a red blood cell count of 2.82×10^{12}/L, a hemoglobin concentration of 85 g/L, a platelet count of 189×10^9/L, a mean corpuscular volume of 88.3 fl, a mean corpuscular hemoglobin content of 30.1 pg, a mean corpuscular hemoglobin concentration of 341 g/L, and a reticulocyte count of 1.06%. His serum iron concentration was 11.3 μmol/L; the total iron-binding rate was 46.7 μmol/L; the transferrin saturation was 24%; and the iron protein concentration was 605.1 μg/L. Moreover, folic acid was 107 μg/L; vitamin B_{12} was 320 pg/ml; erythropoietin was 10.3 U/ml; urea nitrogen was 10.2 mmol/L; creatinine was 218 μmol/L; and uric acid was 0.459 mmol/L. C-reactive protein was 11.7 mg/L, and procalcitonin was 0.07 ng/ml. The β-D-glucan test was negative; tuberculosis infection test was positive; urine red blood cell count was 15.1/μL; urine white blood cell count was 11.9/μL; urine protein was negative, and osmolality was 1.009. Urine transferrin was <2.2 mg/L; α1 microglobulin was 16.0 mg/L; urine IgG was 3.85 mg/L; and urine microalbumin was 12.1 mg/L. Anti-nuclear antibody (ANA), double-stranded DNA (dsDNA), ENA antibody profile, anti-neutrophil cytoplasmic antibody (ANCA), and anti-glomerular basement membrane (GBM) antibodies were all negative. Complement and immunoglobulin panels were normal. The concentration of squamous cell carcinoma-associated antigen was 3.1 ng/mL, and the other tumor parameters were normal. Blood/urine immunofixation electrophoresis found no monoclonal immunoglobulins. Chest CT findings were normal, and there was no evidence of tuberculosis infection. The size of the left kidney was 124 mm × 60 mm, whereas the size of the right kidney was 123 mm × 49 mm; the echogenicity of the bilateral renal parenchyma was high, and there was a left renal cyst. Renal B-mode ultrasound revealed no hepatosplenomegaly.

On admission, the patient had high blood pressure, normal cardiac function, and no allergic reactions. Acute kidney injury (AKI) caused by hypoperfusion was not considered for the time being. The patient had no symptoms of oliguria, hematuria, low back pain, or dysuria, and B-mode ultrasound did not indicate urinary tract obstruction, so we ruled out AKI caused by obstruction for the time being. After excluding contraindications, renal biopsy was performed under the guidance of B ultrasound on March 19, 2019, and the pathological results suggested acute phosphate nephropathy (Figs. 28.1 and 28.2). Considering that the patient had ingested a large amount of phosphate in a short time and the symptoms were mainly chronic, the patient was given Shen Shuai Ning tablets po, 3 tablets/time, 3 times/day. His blood pressure was 163/89 mmHg after admission, and the patient was given antihypertensive treatment (amlodipine 5 mg orally, once a day). The blood pressure was controlled at (110 ~ 100)/(80 ~ 70) mmHg. From March to September 2019, the patient continued to have mild to moderate renal anemia, which was not corrected.

Beginning on September 25, 2019, the patient was followed up at the Chronic Kidney Disease Nutrition Clinic of our hospital and was given 5000 U of EPO

Fig. 28.1 Pathological results of renal biopsy in patients. Note: H&E-stained (200×) dark purple calcium phosphate crystals (yellow arrow) are deposited in the tubules and interstitium

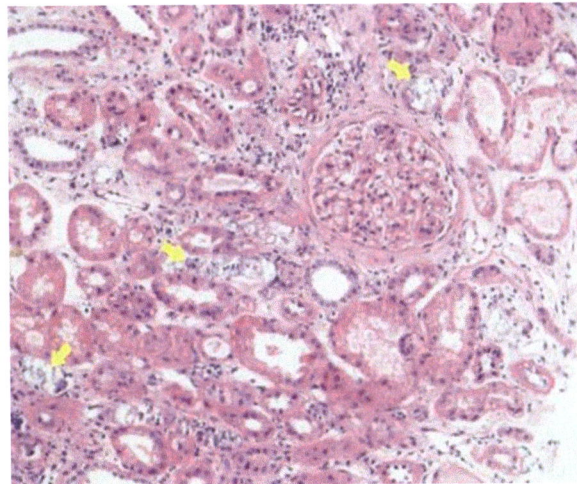

Fig. 28.2 Pathological results of renal biopsy in patients (von Kossa staining). Note: Von Kossa staining (100×) showing black calcium phosphate deposition in renal tissue

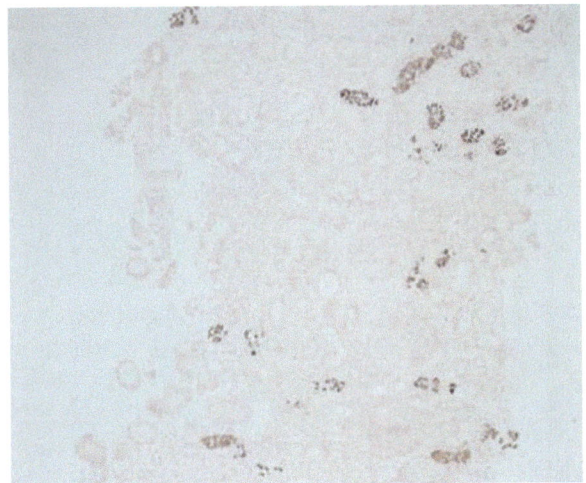

(Erythropoietin) via subcutaneous injection, once a week. On October 31, 2019, the patient was given oral roxadustat at an initial dose of 100 mg three times a week. After 2 months of treatment (December 31, 2019), reexamination revealed a hemoglobin increase ≥ 20 g/L to >120 g/L, and the patient spontaneously reduced his dose of roxadustat to 50 mg three times a week. On January 31, 2020, reexamination showed a hemoglobin concentration of 129 g/L, and the drug was stopped to avoid further increases in hemoglobin. Hemoglobin was not monitored often due to the impact of the COVID-19 epidemic. On February 19, 2020, his hemoglobin was 111 g/L; roxadustat treatment was resumed at a dosage of 50 mg three times a week (Fig. 28.3), and the patient continued regular follow-up in the outpatient clinic.

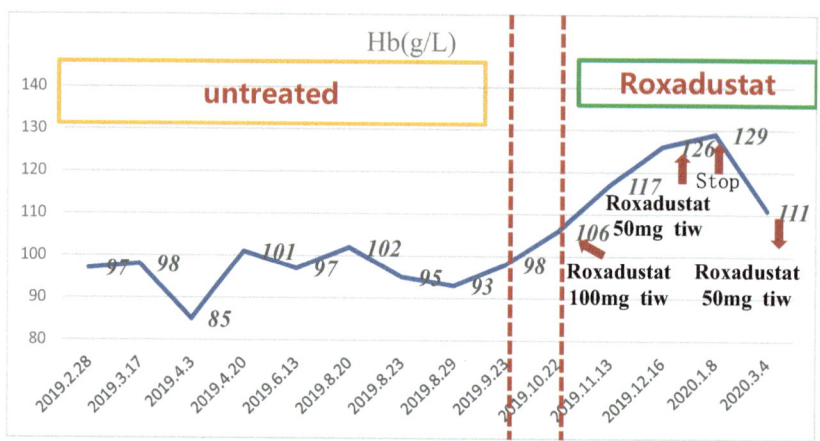

Fig. 28.3 Changes in hemoglobin levels after oral administration of roxadustat. Note: On October 31, 2019, the patient was given roxadustat 100 mg three times/week; on December 31, 2019, the patient spontaneously reduced his dose of roxadustat to 50 mg three times/week; on January 31, 2020, roxadustat was discontinued; on February 29, 2020, roxadustat was resumed at 50 mg three times/week

28.2   Discussion

Acute phosphate nephropathy is one of the less common causes of AKI and is caused by massive phosphate deposition in the renal tubules. Excessive intake of phosphate, early PTH after renal transplantation, and hypophosphatemic rickets in children can cause excessively high intratubular phosphate concentration, especially in patients with a history of CKD or who have used drugs affecting renal blood perfusion. In patients who receive large amounts of sodium phosphate for bowel preparation, the probability of acute phosphate nephropathy ranges from 1 in 5000 to 1 in 1000 [1]. The direct cause of acute phosphate nephropathy in this patient was the administration of sodium phosphate, which resulted in the accumulation of phosphate in the renal tubules. ARBs may increase the risk of AKI. Renal injury due to oral sodium phosphate includes recent acute phosphate nephropathy and remote CKD [2]. The mechanism of renal injury induced by phosphate may be related to the immune response activated by crystal deposition and further induction of the inflammatory response. It has been suggested that phosphate can induce the release of inflammatory factors and cellular oxidative stress damage [3]. Research indicates that renal biopsies conducted four months after enteroscopy in patients with acute kidney injury (AKI) related to oral sodium phosphate intake reveal tubular injury in all examined renal biopsy specimens. These specimens also exhibited tubular atrophy and interstitial fibrosis; glomerulosclerosis was present in a subset of the samples. After 16 months of follow-up, creatinine levels did not return to pre-injury levels in any of the patients (the mean creatinine value was 211 μmol/L). Some patients even progressed to the need for hemodialysis. The stage of end-stage renal disease (ESRD) of the intervention was analyzed [2].

AKI is increasingly recognized as an important factor leading to ESRD, as approximately 6% of AKI patients progress to ESRD within 2 years of diagnosis [4]. AKI has also been found to cause irreversible renal function damage and structural changes, such as tubulointerstitial fibrosis and capillary rarefaction, in animal models. The key mediator of cellular adaptation to hypoxia is hypoxia-inducible factor (HIF), which is regulated by dioxygenases containing prolyl 4-hydroxylase domains [5]. Although the activation of HIF prevents ischemic cell death, HIF has been shown to promote fibrosis in experimental models of CKD [6, 7]. Kapitsinou et al. reported that inhibition of HIF prolyl hydroxylation before AKI improved fibrosis and prevented anemia, whereas inhibition of HIF prolyl hydroxylation during the early recovery phase of AKI did not affect short- or long-term clinical outcomes [8].

The current patient developed AKI due to acute phosphate poisoning and developed CKD, renal insufficiency, concurrent mild to moderate renal anemia, and tubulointerstitial nephritis. Roxadustat corrected his anemia and improved his renal function to some extent. Early administration of HIF-PHI improves the symptoms of renal interstitial fibrosis in CKD rats and may effectively improve renal function [8]. However, this finding is limited to animal models. Clinical trials with longer observation periods are needed to assess the effect of early treatment with HIF-PHI on the improvement of renal function in patients with interstitial nephritis.

This case illustrates the clinical presentation, diagnosis, and successful management of acute phosphate nephropathy by roxadustat. This case underscores the importance of considering the diagnosis of acute phosphate nephropathy in patients with sudden renal function deterioration following exposure to risk factors such as oral sodium phosphate. The use of roxadustat in treating renal anemia in the context of CKD was also discussed, along with its mechanism of action and clinical benefits.

References

1. Fogo AB, et al. AJKD Atlas of Renal Pathology: Nephrocalcinosis and Acute Phosphate Nephropathy. Am J Kidney Dis. 2017;69(3):e17–8.
2. Markowitz GS, et al. Acute phosphate nephropathy following oral sodium phosphate bowel purgative: an underrecognized cause of chronic renal failure. J Am Soc Nephrol. 2005;16(11):3389–96.
3. Yamada Y, et al. Acute phosphate nephropathy with diffuse tubular injury despite limited calcium phosphate deposition. Intern Med. 2016;55(16):2229–35.
4. Lo LJ, et al. Dialysis-requiring acute renal failure increases the risk of progressive chronic kidney disease. Kidney Int. 2009;76(8):893–9.
5. Fu Q, Colgan SP, Shelley CS. Hypoxia: the force that drives chronic kidney disease. Clin Med Res. 2016;14(1):15–39.
6. Li H, et al. Interactions between HIF-1α and AMPK in the regulation of cellular hypoxia adaptation in chronic kidney disease. Am J Physiol Renal Physiol. 2015;309(5):F414–28.
7. Kobayashi H, et al. Myeloid cell-derived hypoxia-inducible factor attenuates inflammation in unilateral ureteral obstruction-induced kidney injury. J Immunol. 2012;188(10):5106–15.
8. Kapitsinou PP, et al. Preischemic targeting of HIF prolyl hydroxylation inhibits fibrosis associated with acute kidney injury. Am J Physiol Renal Physiol. 2012;302(9):F1172–9.

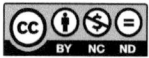

One Case of Peritoneal Dialysis Complicated with Refractory Hypertension and Renal Anemia

Rong-rong Hu, Hai-yun Wang, and Xue-mei Li

29.1 Case Presentation

We presented a 52-year-old male patient. He was followed up by our peritoneal dialysis center for elevated blood pressure for 36 years and peritoneal dialysis for more than 9 years.

In 1984, he was diagnosed with hypertension with blood pressure 170/110 mmHg during physical examination, without dizziness, headache, blurred vision, or nausea. He had no palpitations, wheezing, lower limb edema, or other symptoms of discomfort. Routine blood test and urinalysis showed no significant abnormalities. He did not regularly monitor his blood pressure. In 1990, his blood pressure increased to 220/180 mmHg without obvious symptoms. Metoprolol 25 mg twice a day and nifedipine 20 mg twice a day were prescribed. His blood pressure fluctuated around 130/90 mmHg; his serum creatinine was within the normal range; his urine protein was negative, and urine occult blood test (++), without regular monitoring. In early 2011, the patient experienced wheezing after climbing one floor or walking 50 m on flat ground, which was associated with palpitations, sweating, and mild pitting edema of both lower limbs. Discomfort such as paroxysmal nocturnal dyspnea, anuria, cough, or sputum was not reported. In September 2011, he visited another hospital, where his serum creatinine was reported high as 2200 μmol/L. He was referred to our emergency department. After temporary hemodialysis treatment, he preferred peritoneal dialysis for long-term replacement therapy. In November 2011, he started maintenance peritoneal dialysis treatment after peritoneal dialysis tube implantation.

In May 2017, the patient progressed from regular continuous ambulatory peritoneal dialysis to intermittent peritoneal dialysis. His peritoneal dialysis prescription was four exchanges/day; his ultrafiltration volume was about 1200 ml/d, and his

R.-r. Hu · H.-y. Wang · X.-m. Li (✉)
Department of Nephrology, Peking Union Medical College Hospital, Chinese Academy of Medical Sciences, Beijing, China

© The Author(s) 2025
B.-C. Liu (ed.), *Treatment of Refractory Renal Anemia*,
https://doi.org/10.1007/978-981-97-7636-8_29

Kt/V was 1.83. The patient's dry weight was 71 kg. His other conditions were as follows: (1) Hypertension, for which he took olmesartan 20 mg twice a day, felodipine 5 mg twice a day, arotinolol hydrochloride tablets 15 mg twice a day, amlodipine 5 mg once a day, and doxazosin 8 mg once a night. His blood pressure was about 130/80 mmHg in recent years. (2) Chronic kidney disease–mineral-bone disorder (CKD-MBD), for which he took calcium carbonate 1000 mg, chewed during meals 3 times/day, and sevelamer 3.2 g three times/day. His serum calcium was 2.45 mmol/L, serum phosphorus 1.98 mmol/L, and parathyroid hormone 212 pg/ml. (3) Blood lipids: his low-density lipoprotein cholesterol was 2.53 mmol/L, total cholesterol 4.16 mmol/L, and triglycerides 1.59 mmol/L without drug intervention. (4) Nutritional indicators: his serum albumin was 33 g/L, prealbumin 339 mg/L, and standardized protein breakdown rate (nPCR) 0.89 g/(kg·d). (5) Renal anemia, for which he took ferrous succinate tablets 0.2 g three times/day and subcutaneous injection of erythropoiesis-stimulating agent (ESA), dosed according to the hemoglobin level. His ESA dose in the past year was 10,000 U/week, and his hemoglobin was 96 ~ 136 g/L. His ferritin was 391 μg/L, serum iron 10.6 μmol/L, and transferrin saturation 24.5%. (6) Liver function, alanine aminotransferase, and bilirubin were normal.

The patient denied smoking, and he drank 100 ~ 150 ml of liquor two to three times a month. No remarkable past medical history or family medical history was recorded.

He was 167 cm tall. His blood pressure was 133/81 mmHg. His heart rate was 81 beats/min with a regular rhythm. No crackles or wheezing was heard in either lung. The abdomen was soft but not tender. There was no edema in either lower limb, and no exudate or skin redness or swelling was observed at the exit of the peritoneal dialysis catheter.

Before he was prescribed roxadustat, routine blood tests revealed a red blood cell count of $3.81 \times 10^{12}/L$, hemoglobin of 112 g/L, mean corpuscular volume of 88.2 fl, mean corpuscular hemoglobin of 29.4 pg, mean corpuscular hemoglobin concentration of 333 g/L, white blood cell count of $8.63 \times 10^9/L$, and platelet count of $223 \times 10^9/L$. An iron metabolism test revealed that his serum iron concentration was 10.6 μmol/L, total iron-binding capacity was 241 μg/dL, transferrin concentration was 1.71 g/L, transferrin saturation was 24.5%, and ferritin concentration was 391 μg/L.

This patient's weight was 71 kg. Renal replacement therapy, anemia correction, and blood pressure control were continued. During anemia treatment, he changed to oral administration of roxadustat (120 mg) three times a week. Ferrous succinate tablets were continued. The medication intervals between the sevelamer, calcium

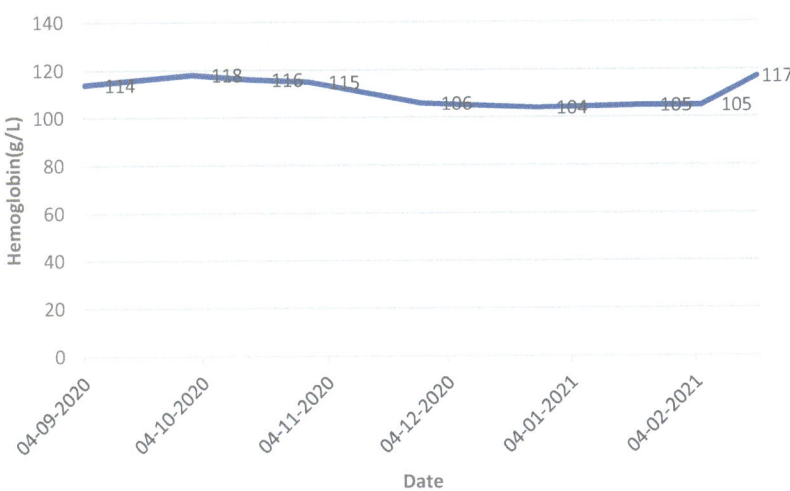

Fig. 29.1 Hemoglobin level during treatment of roxadustat. Note: From September 4 to September 30, 2020, the patient received roxadustat 120 mg, tid; from October 1 to December 25, 2020, the patient received roxadustat 100 mg, tid; from December 26, 2020 to February 4, 2021, the patient received roxadustat 120 mg, tid; from February 5 to 19, 2021, the patient received roxadustat 150 mg, tid

carbonate, and roxadustat treatments were greater than 1 hour. Then, his hemoglobin levels were closely monitored, and the dose of roxadustat was adjusted according to the change in hemoglobin (Fig. 29.1).

From October to December 2020, the patient's hemoglobin decreased, his appetite and diet did not change substantially; no gastrointestinal bleeding was detected, and fecal occult blood was negative. The patient's parathyroid hormone level increased to 1113.8 pg/ml, and after adjusting his CKD-MBD treatment, his hemoglobin level turned to normal, and the hemoglobin fluctuation was considered normal relative to the high parathyroid hormone.

Changes in clinical parameters such as blood pressure were monitored during the administration of roxadustat (Table 29.1). We found that amlodipine could be discontinued after one month of roxadustat administration. As the dosage of doxazosin gradually decreased, his blood pressure stayed within (110 ~ 120)/(70 ~ 80) mmHg. Under the same oral iron supplementation, his serum iron increased and ferritin decreased. During this time, the patient had no nausea, vomiting, diarrhea, abdominal discomfort, or other adversed reactions.

Table 29.1 Changes in iron metabolism, blood lipids, nutrition, and blood pressure while taking roxadustat

Item		Baseline	One month after treatment	Two months after treatment
Iron metabolism index	Serum iron (μmol/L)	8.8	8.3	16.0
	Total iron-binding capacity (μmol/L)	38.2	50.7	47.2
	Transferrin (g/L)	1.84	1.99	1.86
	Transferrin saturation (%)	23.00	16.40	33.90
	Ferritin (μg/L)	298.51	308.00	268.00
Lipids	Total cholesterol (mmol/L)	2.29	2.00	1.69
	Triglyceride (mmol/L)	0.61	0.67	0.35
	High-density lipoprotein (mmol/L)	1.11	1.00	0.89
	Low-density lipoprotein (mmol/L)	0.91	0.59	0.58
Nutritional indicators	Serum albumin (g/L)	32	32	33
	Prealbumin (mg/L)	336	349	388
Blood pressure (mmHg)		133/81	133/72	99/72[a]

Note: [a]During this follow-up, the patient's blood pressure was low, so the dose of antihypertensive drugs was reduced

29.2 Discussion

Here, we presented a case of a middle-aged man who had early-onset hypertension that was not well controlled. He eventually progressed to end-stage renal disease (ESRD). Peritoneal dialysis was chosen for long-term renal placement because hemodialysis was unavailable near his home. He suffered from complications of ESRD, such as CKD-MBD and renal anemia. The anemia could be corrected with oral iron and subcutaneous ESA, but his hypertension was difficult to control, and up to five antihypertensive drugs were needed. Luckily, after treatment with roxadustat, not only renal anemia was well corrected, but blood pressure control became easy, and two of his antihypertensive drugs were reduced or discontinued.

In this patient with refractory hypertension, blood pressure control significantly improved during treatment with roxadustat instead of ESA. In a phase III clinical study of roxadustat in China, blood pressure decreased more in the roxadustat group than in the ESA group, but the difference was not statistically significant [1]. The mechanism of blood pressure regulation by roxadustat is not yet clear. During phase II clinical studies of roxadustat in maintenance hemodialysis patients, Robert et al. [2] reported that EPO concentrations fluctuated less in patients receiving oral roxadustat than in those receiving intravenous EPO. However, their study did not compare the changes in patients' blood pressure, so it is hard to say whether the improvement in blood pressure control was related to the small wave of EPO in vivo.

Because the HIF-mediated transcriptional cascade includes a series of genes involved in vasomotor regulation, HIF-PHI may regulate blood pressure through vasomotor regulation. In an angiotensin II (Ang II)-induced hypertension model, Jing Yu, et al. showed that FG-4592 abolished hypertensive responses and prevented vascular thickening, cardiac hypertrophy, and kidney injury by downregulating Angiotensin II Receptor Type 1 (AGTR1) expression and enhancing expression of AGTR2 and endothelial NO synthase (eNOS) [3]. Another HIF-PHI, that is, molidustat, could also significantly reduce the systolic blood pressure in rats, and this effect may be related to its regulation of prorenin concentration [4].

Roxadustat is metabolized mainly through UDP-glucuronosyltransferases (UGT) 1A9 and cytochrome P450 proteins (CYP)2C8 [5]. We also checked the patient's antihypertensives and ruled out the interaction between roxadustat and antihypertensives. Thus, the good blood pressure control with roxadustat in this patient may not be due to its influence on the action of other antihypertensives, but rather to the fact that roxadustat may have antihypertensive effects.

Roxadustat provides an alternative treatment option for maintenance dialysis patients due to its effectiveness in correcting anemia, and it is more convenient [5]. During the treatment of our patient, roxadustat helped improve his refractory hypertension and simplified his antihypertensive treatment. Large-scale clinical studies are needed to determine whether roxadustat can improve hypertension control. The underlying mechanism also needs to be further explored.

References

1. Chen N, Hao C, Liu BC, et al. Roxadustat treatment for anemia in patients undergoing long-term dialysis. N Engl J Med. 2019;381(11):1011–22.
2. Provenzano R, Besarab A, Wright S, et al. Roxadustat (FG-4592) versus epoetin alfa for anemia in patients receiving maintenance hemodialysis: a phase 2, randomized, 6- to 19-week, open-label, active-comparator, dose-ranging, safety and exploratory efficacy study. Am J Kidney Dis. 2016;67(6):912–24.
3. Jing Y, Wang S, Shi W, et al. Roxadustat prevents Ang II hypertension by targeting angiotensin receptors and eNOS. JCI Insight. 2021;6(18):e133690.
4. Flamme I, Oehme F, Ellinghaus P, Jeske M, Keldenich J, Thuss U. Mimicking hypoxia to treat anemia: HIF-stabilizer BAY 85-3934 (Molidustat) stimulates erythropoietin production without hypertensive effects. PLoS One. 2014;9(11):e111838.
5. Liu Q, Xu Y, Wang L, et al. Investigation on the compliance of using erythropoietin in peritoneal dialysis patients. Chin J Mod Nurs. 2010;34:4131–2.

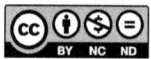

Effect of Roxadustat on Glucose and Lipid Metabolism in a Patient with Renal Anemia on Peritoneal Dialysis

30

Chunli-Cui and Chen-Yu

30.1 Case Presentation

30.1.1 History of Present Illness

A 33-year-old male patient was diagnosed with IgA nephropathy 3 years ago and had been on peritoneal dialysis for more than a year. He was admitted to the hospital for further evaluation. On April 12, 2018, the patient was admitted to the endocrinology department of our hospital due to type 2 diabetes. Laboratory test showed as follows: 24-h urinary protein, 12.93 g; HLA-B27, positive; creatinine, 143 μmol/L; eGFR, 53.4 mL/min; uric acid, 477 μmol/L; and albumin, 30.2 g/L.

Renal biopsy was performed on April 24, 2018, and he was diagnosed as "IgA nephropathy with renal arteriosclerosis." As a result, prednisone and cyclophosphamide were initiated as part of his treatment. However, there was no significant improvement in his proteinuria, and the patient's blood glucose and blood pressure remained poorly controlled throughout the disease. Additionally, a progressive increase in creatinine levels was observed. On May 26, 2020, the patient underwent peritoneal dialysis catheterization under local anesthesia. Since then, he had been on peritoneal dialysis. His current peritoneal dialysis regimen involves continuous ambulatory peritoneal dialysis (CAPD) with 2.5% peritoneal dialysis solution (4 packets), resulting in approximately 1000 mL of daily ultrafiltration and 100–200 mL of urinary production. Roxadustat is administered during the peritoneal dialysis period to address anemia, and atorvastatin is used to manage lipid metabolism disorder, among other measures. On October 24, 2021, the patient was readmitted for peritoneal dialysis assessment.

Chunli-Cui · Chen-Yu (✉)
Department of Nephrology, Tongji Hospital, School of Medicine, Tongji University, Shanghai, China
e-mail: yuchne@tongji.edu.cnn

© The Author(s) 2025
B.-C. Liu (ed.), *Treatment of Refractory Renal Anemia*,
https://doi.org/10.1007/978-981-97-7636-8_30

30.1.2 History of Past Illness

The patient had over 5-year history of ankylosing spondylitis for which he had been prescribed oral sulfasalazine (0.75 g, three times daily) for long-term treatment. Additionally, the patient had been diagnosed with type 2 diabetes mellitus for more than 3 years and had been using insulin as part of the treatment for an extended duration. However, for the past 6 months, the patient has not required insulin therapy and has maintained good control of his blood glucose levels. Furthermore, the patient had been diagnosed with hypertension for more than 2 years, with a maximum recorded blood pressure of 220/100 mmHg. Currently, the patient is taking a combination of orally administered medications, including aronixil, amlodipine, doxazosin, and sacubitril/valsartan, for hypertension management. The patient has a long-standing history of hyperuricemia for which he had been prescribed 40 mg of febuxostat once daily. The patient denied any history of hepatitis, tuberculosis, malaria, cardiac disease, cerebrovascular disease, mental illness, surgery, trauma, blood transfusion, food allergies, or drug allergies. Additionally, the patient's vaccination history was available locally.

30.1.3 Family Medical History

The patient denied a family history of genetic or infectious diseases.

30.1.4 Physical Examination at Admission

The patient's vital signs were as follows: body temperature (T), 36.0 °C; pulse (P), 80 beats/minute; respiration (R), 18 breaths/minute; blood pressure (BP), 160/80 mmHg; and body mass index (BMI), 25.

On examination, there were no signs of xanthochromia on the skin mucosa throughout the body, and the superficial lymph nodes were neither palpable nor enlarged. The jugular vein showed no signs of dilation, and the thyroid gland was not tender upon palpation. Auscultation of the lungs revealed clear breath sounds without any dry or wet rales. During cardiac boundary percussion, the heart rate was recorded as 80 beats/minute, and the rhythm was regular. No pathological murmurs were detected. Abdominal examination revealed a soft and nontender abdomen without any rebound pain or bulges. There was no exudation at the outlet of the abdominal transit duct, and the liver and spleen were not enlarged. Moreover, the lower limb showed no signs of edema.

30.1.5 Supplementary Examination

On October 26, 2021, the patient's glycated hemoglobin and fasting blood glucose levels were normal. The parathyroid hormone level (PTH) was 1340 pg/mL;

the ferritin level was 324 ng/mL; the vitamin B12 level was 1329 pmol/L; and the folic acid level was 3.84 ng/mL. The routine blood test results were as follows: hemoglobin (Hb), 92 g/L; red blood cell (RBC) count, 3.05 × 1012/L; white blood cell (WBC) count, 11.19 × 10^9/L; platelet (PLT) count, 288 × 10^9/L; and neutrophil (N) count, 8.8 × 10^9/L. Blood biochemical parameters were as follows: albumin, 38 g/L; creatinine, 1037 μmol/L; uric acid, 607 μmol/L; urea, 29.1 mmol/L; total cholesterol, 6.23 mmol/L; triglyceride, 2.31 mmol/L; potassium, 3.18 mmol/L; phosphorus, 2.97 mmol/L; total calcium, 2.22 mmol/L; and chlorine, 92.3 mmol/L. Urinary protein quantification results were as follows: volume, 100 mL (1000–1500 mL); total urinary protein (24 h), 0.62 g/24 h (0.028 g/24 h-0.14 g/24 h); and β2 microglobulin, 43.00 mg/L (2.8 mg/L). Positron emission tomography (PET) showed high average transport, with a KT/V of 1.66. B-scan ultrasound revealed no obvious abnormalities in the bilateral upper limbs.

30.1.6 Clinical Diagnosis

1. IgA nephropathy, peritoneal dialysis, renal anemia, and chronic kidney disease-mineral bone disorder (CKD-MBD)
2. Type 2 diabetes and diabetic retinopathy
3. Hyperuricemia
4. Hypertensive disease grade 3 (extremely high risk)
5. Ankylosing spondylitis

30.2 Clinical Treatment Process

A 33-year-old male patient commenced maintenance peritoneal dialysis in May 2020. His medical regimen has included active management of blood glucose with insulin, along with the administration of sacubitril/valsartan, amlodipine, and Alprolix for blood pressure control, lipid regulation, plaque stabilization, anemia correction, mineral metabolism disorder correction, and uric acid reduction. The patient initiated roxadustat treatment following the insertion of a peritoneal dialysis catheter on May 26, 2020. Subsequent to the commencement of roxadustat therapy and continuation of peritoneal dialysis, the patient exhibited a progressive increase in hemoglobin levels, reaching 120 g/L by September 9, 2020 and further rising to 124 g/L by October 26, 2020 (Fig. 30.1). During the course of treatment, a notable adjustment was observed in the patient's atorvastatin dosage, which was reduced from an initial 20 mg per day to 10 mg per day (Fig. 30.2). Furthermore, the patient's insulin requirement significantly decreased, culminating in the discontinuation of insulin therapy in May 2021 (Fig. 30.3). A reduction in the patient's BMI was also recorded (Fig. 30.4). No adverse reactions were reported throughout the treatment period. However, the patient's adherence to the prescribed treatment regimen was suboptimal, characterized by irregular medication intake and unsupervised dosage adjustments. This noncompliance has potentially impacted the overall therapeutic efficacy.

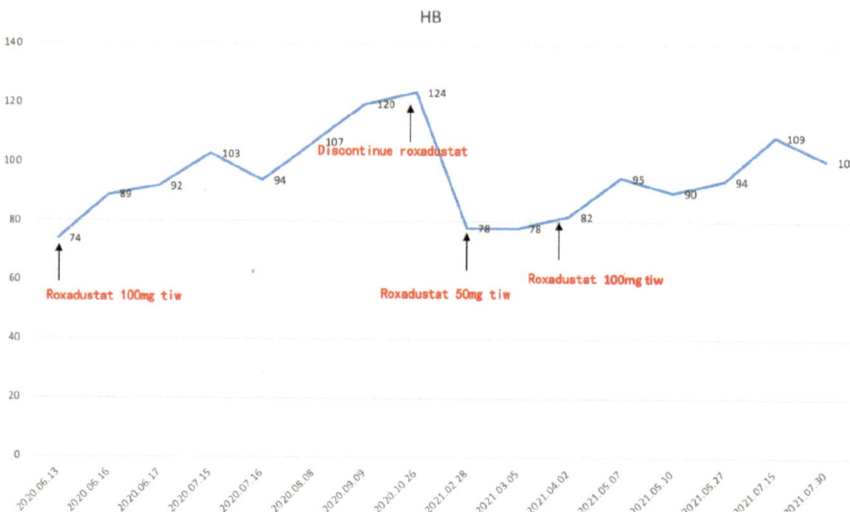

Fig. 30.1 Changes in patient hemoglobin levels during treatment 纵坐标要标出单位(如 Hemoglobin, g/L)

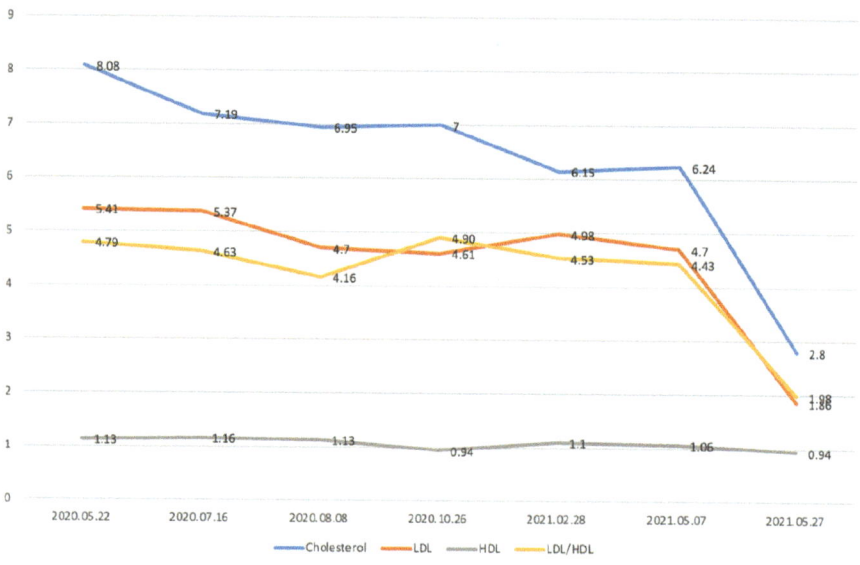

Fig. 30.2 Changes in blood cholesterol, low-density lipoprotein (LDL), high-density lipoprotein (HDL), and LDL/HDL during treatment

This case highlights the efficacy of roxadustat in conjunction with peritoneal dialysis and other supportive therapies in managing anemia and associated metabolic conditions in a patient with chronic kidney disease. Nonetheless, patient compliance remains a critical factor in the success of the therapeutic regimen. Further emphasis on patient education and adherence strategies is warranted to optimize clinical outcomes.

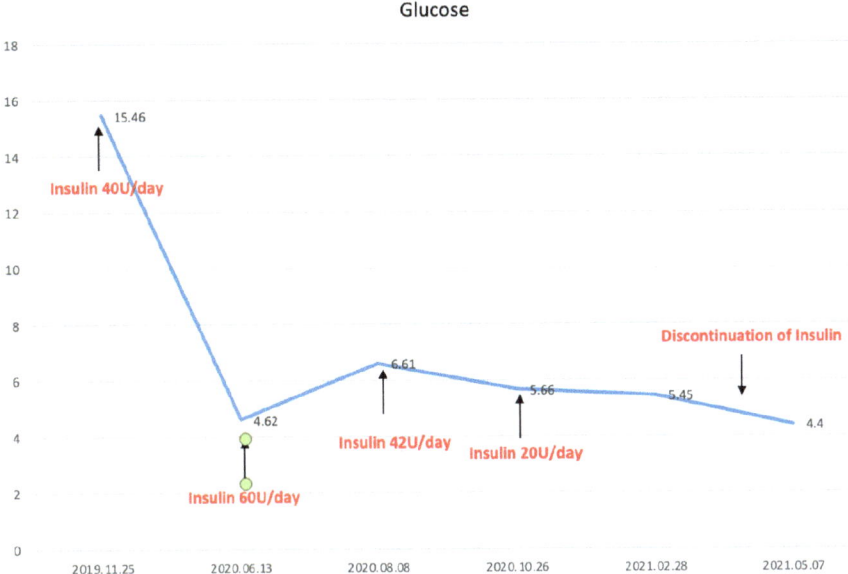

Fig. 30.3   Changes in patient blood glucose during treatment

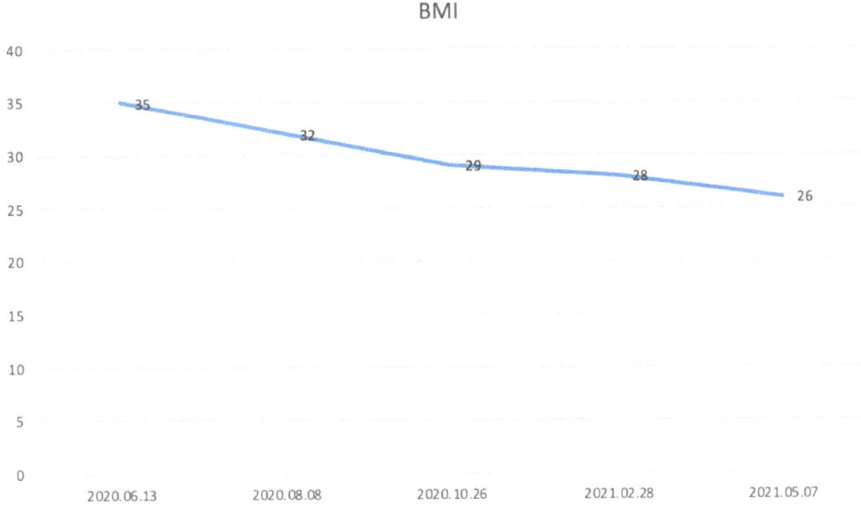

Fig. 30.4   Changes in patient BMI during treatment

30.3   Discussion

Here, we reported a case of a patient with chronic kidney disease who underwent peritoneal dialysis with renal anemia. He was treated with roxadustat, and his Hb levels successfully increased to 124 g after the treatment (Fig. 30.1). The patient had a fluctuated Hb when he stopped or reduced the dosage of the drug. These findings indicate the efficacy of roxadustat in this patient and further emphasize the importance for close monitoring and appropriated dosage adjustments during the treatment of renal anemia.

Interestingly, the patient's glycemic control improved while on roxadustat (Fig. 30.3). Subsequently, insulin treatment was discontinued due to hypoglycemia, a rare occurrence in diabetic patients on peritoneal dialysis. Previous study suggests that long-term exposure to glucose contributes to an increased incidence of diabetes. Many diabetic patients require higher insulin doses after poor blood glucose control, or they may develop metabolic syndrome. This diabetic patient undergoing peritoneal dialysis was able to control blood glucose without insulin treatment after using roxadustat. There are currently no reports linking this to the use of roxadustat; thus, this mechanism deserves further observation.

Furthermore, this patient experienced a decrease in BMI after treatment with roxadustat (Fig. 30.4). And his dosage of atorvastatin also reduced but maintained a decrease in cholesterol levels, low-density lipoprotein cholesterol (LDL), and the LDL-to-high-density lipoprotein cholesterol (HDL) ratio. We followed up the patient for 1 year and found that there was a significant improvement in the patient's lipid metabolism and glucose metabolism disorders, which induced his insulin and resulted in other hypoglycemic drugs no longer in use.

Roxadustat (FG-4592; ASP1517; AZD9941) is an oral hypoxia-inducing factor prolyl hydroxylase inhibitor that stimulates erythropoiesis, enhances iron utilization, and corrects renal anemia [1, 2]. Clinical application of roxadustat in treating chronic kidney disease (CKD)-related anemia has shown a notable reduction in cholesterol levels, although the underlying mechanism remains incompletely understood. Currently, three potential pathways are proposed:

1. Increased stability of HIF-1α and elevated mRNA levels of insulin-inducible gene 2 (INSIG2) in the liver promote the degradation of HMG-CoA reductase and inhibit cholesterol synthesis. Insulin has been shown to enhance HMG-CoA reductase activity. Therefore, when PHD2 inhibition reduces serum insulin levels, HMG-CoA reductase activity decreases, subsequently reducing hepatic cholesterol synthesis [3, 4].
2. Increased expression of HIF-1α and HIF-2α in the liver leads to a downregulation of fat synthesis genes and an upregulation of lipolysis genes through a Srebp-1c-dependent pathway, thereby increasing fat metabolism [5, 6].
3. Increased expression of HIF-2α in adipocytes upregulates the downstream target gene ACER2. ACER2 reduces ceramide levels, subsequently increasing the expression of cholesterol elimination genes (Cp7a1, Abcg5/8), reducing liver and plasma cholesterol levels, and promoting adipose tissue thermogenesis, resulting in reductions in lipid levels [7].
4. HIF improves insulin secretion and resistance through IRS2 and promotes the expression of glucose transporters (GLUT-1,3), facilitating glucose entry into cells [7, 8]. More importantly, it changes the intracellular metabolism, favoring glucose entry into the anaerobic glycolytic pathway to reduce the mitochondrial damage caused by glucose entry into mitochondrial metabolism pathways.

Stable intracellular HIF under hypoxia initiates alterations in cell metabolism. For example, HIF-1 induces the expression of pyruvate dehydrogenase kinase (PDK), leading to inactivation of PDK phosphorylation, inhibition of pyruvate conversion into acetyl-CoA for the tricarboxylic acid cycle (TCA) cycle, reduction in oxidative phosphorylation in mitochondria, and decrease in superoxide production. HIF-1 also promotes increased lactate synthesis through transcriptional activation of lactate dehydrogenase, enhancing glycolysis [9, 10].

This interesting case demonstrated that roxadustat could not only improve renal anemia, but also reduce blood cholesterol, LDL levels, and the BMI as well as correct diabetes, suggesting the unique potential role of this drug in managing glucose and lipid metabolism disorders. However, due to the limited clinical observation, further investigation is warranted to elucidate its underlying mechanisms.

References

1. Chen N, Qian J, Chen J, Yu X, Mei C, Hao C, Jiang G, Lin H, Zhang X, Zuo L, He Q, Fu P, Li X, Ni D, Hemmerich S, Liu C, Szczech L, Besarab A, Neff TB, Peony Yu KH, Valone FH. Phase 2 studies of oral hypoxia-inducible factor prolyl hydroxylase inhibitor FG-4592 for treatment of anemia in China. Nephrol Dial Transplant. 2017;32(8):1373–86.
2. Chen N, Hao C, Liu BC, Lin H, Wang C, Xing C, Liang X, Jiang G, Liu Z, Li X, Zuo L, Luo L, Wang J, Zhao MH, Liu Z, Cai GY, Hao L, Leong R, Wang C, Liu C, Neff T, Szczech L, Yu KP. Roxadustat treatment for anemia in patients undergoing long-term dialysis. N Engl J Med. 2019;381(11):1011–22.
3. Pallottini V, Guantario B, Martini C, Totta P, Filippi I, Carraro F, Trentalance A. Regulation of HMG-CoA reductase expression by hypoxia. J Cell Biochem. 2008;104(3):701–9.
4. Hwang S, Nguyen AD, Jo Y, Engelking LJ, Brugarolas J, DeBose-Boyd RA. Hypoxia-inducible factor 1α activates insulin-induced gene 2 (Insig-2) transcription for degradation of 3-hydroxy-3-methylglutaryl (HMG)-CoA reductase in the liver. J Biol Chem. 2017;292(22):9382–93.
5. Liu Y, Ma Z, Zhao C, Wang Y, Wu G, Xiao J, McClain CJ, Li X, Feng W. HIF-1α and HIF-2α are critically involved in hypoxia-induced lipid accumulation in hepatocytes through reducing PGC-1α-mediated fatty acid β-oxidation. Toxicol Lett. 2014;226(2):117–23.
6. Nishiyama Y, Goda N, Kanai M, Niwa D, Osanai K, Yamamoto Y, Senoo-Matsuda N, Johnson RS, Miura S, Kabe Y, Suematsu M. HIF-1α induction suppresses excessive lipid accumulation in alcoholic fatty liver in mice. J Hepatol. 2012;56(2):441–7.
7. Rahtu-Korpela L, Karsikas S, Hörkkö S, Blanco Sequeiros R, Lammentausta E, Mäkelä KA, Herzig KH, Walkinshaw G, Kivirikko KI, Myllyharju J, Serpi R, Koivunen P. HIF prolyl 4-hydroxylase-2 inhibition improves glucose and lipid metabolism and protects against obesity and metabolic dysfunction. Diabetes. 2014;63(10):3324–33.
8. Goda N, Kanai M. Hypoxia-inducible factors and their roles in energy metabolism. Int J Hematol. 2012;95(5):457–63.
9. Semba H, Takeda N, Isagawa T, Sugiura Y, Honda K, Wake M, Miyazawa H, Yamaguchi Y, Miura M, Jenkins DM, Choi H, Kim JW, Asagiri M, Cowburn AS, Abe H, Soma K, Koyama K, Katoh M, Sayama K, Goda N, Komuro I. HIF-1α-PDK1 axis-induced active glycolysis plays an essential role in macrophage migratory capacity. Nat Commun. 2016;7:11635.
10. Hasegawa S, Tanaka T, Saito T, Fukui K, Wakashima T, Susaki EA, Ueda HR, Nangaku M. The oral hypoxia-inducible factor prolyl hydroxylase inhibitor enarodustat counteracts alterations in renal energy metabolism in the early stages of diabetic kidney disease. Kidney Int. 2020;97(5):934–50.

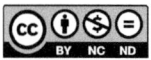

Roxadustat in the Treatment of Renal Anemia in a Hemodialysis Patient

31

XiaoMing Liu, Tao Wang, and LiHong Zhang

31.1 Case Presentation

A 49-year-old female was diagnosed with "diabetic nephropathy" 10 years ago because of foamy urine and edema of both lower limbs. One year prior to admission, the patient was hospitalized again due to nausea, vomiting, and shortness of breath. After completing the relevant examinations, the patient was diagnosed with stage V diabetic nephropathy. During hospitalization, the right femoral vein was catheterized, and hemodialysis treatment was initiated, with a frequency of dialysis of thrice a week. At the same time, a left forearm artificial arteriovenous fistula was generated. The patient's hemoglobin was 80 g/L.

This patient had a 20-year history of diabetes. At present, she was treated with "insulin aspart injection and insulin glargine injection," and her blood sugar is stably controlled. She had a 10-year history of hypertension and regularly used amlodipine besylate tablets and sacubitril valsartan sodium tablets for treatment. Before dialysis, her blood pressure was controlled at approximately 140/80 mmHg. In addition, she had a 3-year history of coronary atherosclerotic heart disease and a 2-year history of Sjogren's syndrome. No other special information regarding her personal or family history was noted.

In the physical examination, her body weight is 65 kg with 1.6 m in height. She had an anemic appearance, pale palpebral conjunctiva, thick respiratory sounds in both lungs, palpable wet rales, enlarged cardiac boundaries, palpable systolic murmurs in the heart, and severe pitting edema in both lower limbs.

Laboratory test results revealed the following: white blood cell count, 4.7×10^9/L; red blood cell count, 3.55×10^{12}/L; hemoglobin, 80 g/L; platelet count, 212×10^9/L; albumin, 35.6 g/L; blood urea nitrogen, 30.39 mmol/L; creatinine (enzymatic

X. Liu · T. Wang (✉) · L. Zhang (✉)
Department of Nephrology, The First Hospital of HeBei Medical University, ShiJiaZhuang, China
e-mail: wangtao-PI@hebmu.edu.cn; lihong-zhang2602@hebmu.edu.cn

© The Author(s) 2025
B.-C. Liu (ed.), *Treatment of Refractory Renal Anemia*,
https://doi.org/10.1007/978-981-97-7636-8_31

method), 840.2 μmol/L; uric acid, 393.7 μmol/L; β_2 microglobulin, 30.8 mg/L; potassium, 5.08 mmol/L; calcium, 2.30 mmol/L; phosphorus, 1.85 mmol/L; fasting blood sugar, 6.78 mmol/L; C-reactive protein, 0.20 mg/L; parathyroid hormone, 226.9 ng/L; ferritin, 50 μg/L; transferrin saturation, 15%; B-type natriuretic peptide, 2207 pg/mL; and urinary protein, 3+. The patient was positive for anti-Ro-52 antibody and anti-SS-A antibody and weakly positive for antinuclear antibody, with an antinuclear antibody titer of 1:100. Serological test results for tumor markers and infectious diseases (hepatitis B, hepatitis C, syphilis, and human immunodeficiency virus) were negative. In addition, serum protein electrophoresis and immunofixation electrophoresis, as well as urine protein electrophoresis and immunofixation electrophoresis, showed no abnormalities.

In auxiliary examination, cardiac ultrasound indicated pulmonary hypertension (mild) and pericardial effusion. Chest computed tomography (CT) revealed pulmonary edema and pleural effusion.

In terms of treatment, to control blood sugar and blood pressure, we arranged for the patient to undergo hemodialysis treatment three times a week. The main problem with this patient was anemia. Initially, recombinant human erythropoietin (EPO) (3000 IU) was given thrice a week to treat renal anemia. After 1 month of treatment, the patient's hemoglobin did not increase. We tested her ferritin and transferrin saturation and confirmed that the patient had iron deficiency, which was treated with iron transfusion and an increased dose of EPO. Nine months later, the patient complained that her blood pressure tended to increase after each dose of EPO. During these increases, her systolic blood pressure fluctuated between 170 and 180 mmHg, while her diastolic blood pressure fluctuated between 90 and 100 mmHg, and the increases were accompanied by headache symptoms. At this time, the patient's dose of EPO was 18,000 IU/week. However, the patient's hemoglobin remained at 75–85 g/L for 3 months. Therefore, we stopped using EPO and instead administered 100 mg roxadustat three times a week. After treatment, the patient's hemoglobin gradually increased, reaching 110 g/L 6 months later, and her blood pressure stabilized.

31.2 Discussion

This middle-aged woman, who regularly underwent hemodialysis, had a history of diabetes, hypertension, coronary heart disease, and Sjogren's syndrome. In the early stage of dialysis, she experienced moderate anemia, and high-dose EPO combined with iron therapy was given. The patient's anemia did not improve, and she experienced discomfort, such as increased blood pressure and headache, after EPO administration. In response to the abovementioned situation, we adjusted the medication for treating anemia to roxadustat and adjusted the dosage according to the instructions. After 3 months of treatment, the patient's hemoglobin level was effectively maintained at 110 g/L. At this time, the patient's dosage of roxadustat was 100 mg three times a week. In addition, the patient's blood pressure was also relatively stable at approximately 140/80 mmHg.

The combination of EPO and iron has been the main method for treating anemia in dialysis patients. However, in clinical practice, some patients have low reactivity to EPO, and some patients are prone to elevated blood pressure after receiving EPO. For this group of patients, roxadustat will be their new choice to improve anemia. There are studies showing that lower blood pressure was observed in the hypoxia-inducible factor prolyl hydroxylase inhibitor (HIF-PHI) group than in the recombinant human EPO group in a mouse model of renal insufficiency [1]. Clinical studies have shown that anemia in peritoneal dialysis patients treated with roxadustat for 40 weeks had significantly lower systolic blood pressure than the recombinant human EPO group [2]. The exchange of recombinant human EPO for roxadustat was effective in avoiding ESA-associated blood pressure elevation in peritoneal dialysis patients combined with anemia [3]. In hemodialysis patients, mean arterial pressure was lower, and antihypertensive medications were used less in the roxadustat group compared to the EPO group [4].

Iron is widely used in dialysis patients; however, an increasing number of studies have shown that iron overload is common in the dialysis population. Iron overload refers to the excessive deposition of iron in the body, leading to structural damage and dysfunction of important organs (especially the heart, liver, pituitary, pancreas, and joints). Clinical manifestations include heart failure, liver fibrosis, diabetes, infertility, growth and development disorders, and even death.

Roxadustat (FG-4592) is the first approved HIF-PHI for clinical use. In 2018, China took the global lead in completing phase III clinical trials for this new-generation drug with a completely new mechanism of action for the treatment of renal anemia, and roxadustat was officially approved for marketing. Roxadustat has been in clinical application for 5 years, and rich clinical experience has been gained [5].

Roxadustat is a small molecule compound that can reversibly inhibit the activity of PHD, simulate the hypoxic environment of the body, and temporarily and dose-dependently induce the stable expression of HIF, thereby promoting the expression of EPO, the downstream target gene of HIF, inducing erythropoiesis, and alleviating renal anemia. In addition, roxadustat can also reduce the level of HAMP; increase the absorption, transport, and utilization of iron by promoting the expression of EPOR in the body; and comprehensively promote the production of red blood cells with multiple targets [6]. Roxadustat can also increase iron metabolism, reduce the need for intravenous iron use, and reduce the risk of iron overload in dialysis patients [7–9].

Here we report a case of patient with poor response to EPO and was prone to elevated blood pressure after EPO administration. After switching to roxadustat, the patient's anemia was resolved, which suggests that roxadustat offers a new approach for the clinical treatment of renal anemia in patients with poor response to EPO.

References

1. Flamme I, Oehme F, Ellinghaus P, et al. Mimicking hypoxia to treat anemia: HIF-stabilizer BAY 85-3934 (Molidustat) stimulates erythropoietin production without hypertensive effects. PLoS One. 2014;9(11):e111838.
2. Wu T, Qi YY, Ma S, et al. Efficacy of Roxadustat on anemia and residual renal function in patients new to peritoneal dialysis. Renal Failure. 2022;44(1):529–40.
3. Zhao YC, Zhao HP, Wu B, et al. Influence of Roxadustat on blood pressure in peritoneal dialysis patients. Chin J Blood Purif. 2022;21(9):633–7.
4. Wang YD, Zhang YM, Zhang DY, et al. Comparison of the effect of anemia on blood pressure in hemodialysis patients treated with human recombinant erythropoietin and roxarestat. J China-Jpn Friendship Hospital. 2022;36(1):22–24.
5. Dhillon S. Roxadustat: first global approval. Drugs. 2019;79(5):563–72.
6. Li ZL, Tu Y, Liu BC. Treatment of renal anemia with roxadustat: advantages and achievement. Kidney Dis (Basel). 2020;6(2):65–73.
7. Charytan C, Manllo-Karim R, Martin ER, et al. A randomized trial of roxadustat in anemia of kidney failure: SIERRAS study. Kidney Int Rep. 2021;6(7):1829–39.
8. Chen N, Hao C, Liu BC, et al. Roxadustat treatment for anemia in patients undergoing long-term dialysis. N Engl J Med. 2019;381(11):1011–22.
9. Ghoti H, Rachmilewitz EA, Simon-Lopez R, et al. Evidence for tissue iron overload in long-term hemodialysis patients and the impact of withdrawing parenteral iron. Eur J Haematol. 2012;89(1):87–93.

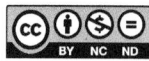

A Patient with Renal Anemia Complicated with Hyperferritinemia

32

Ming-Zhu Li, Yang Zou, and Da-Qing Hong

32.1 Case Presentation

A 70-year-old female presented with a complaint of elevated serum creatinine detected during physical examinations spanning 17 years. In 2003, initial findings revealed elevated serum creatinine levels of approximately 100 μmol/L, along with foamy urine during a physical examination, which indicates chronic renal insufficiency. Oral medications were administered, but the specifics of the treatments were unknown. Regular later examinations showed serum creatinine fluctuating between 100 and 200 μmol/L. By 2014, her serum creatinine had increased to 700 μmol/L, leading to a diagnosis of stage 5 chronic kidney disease. Treatment involved arteriovenous fistuloplasty of the left forearm, followed by thrice-weekly maintenance hemodialysis and subcutaneous administration of rHuEPO at a dosage of 6000 U thrice weekly. Hemoglobin fluctuated between 95 and 120 g/L, accompanied by a notable increase in serum ferritin, peaking at 2721.92 ng/mL. In December 2020, the patient transitioned to outpatient care at a staff hospital for continued hemodialysis treatment.

Over 30 years ago, the patient was diagnosed with hyperthyroidism for which she received pharmacological intervention. After one decade of iodine-131 treatment, the patient's thyroid function decreased, necessitating long-term replacement therapy with levothyroxine sodium (87.5 μg, once daily). Additionally, a history of endoscopic mucosal resection for transverse colon polyps was noted. She had no

M.-Z. Li
Department of Nephrology, The Affiliated Hospital of Southwest Medical University, Luzhou, China

Renal Department and Nephrology Institute, Sichuan Provincial People's Hospital, School of Medicine, University of Electronic Science and Technology of China, Chengdu, China

Y. Zou · D.-Q. Hong (✉)
Renal Department and Nephrology Institute, Sichuan Provincial People's Hospital, School of Medicine, University of Electronic Science and Technology of China, Chengdu, China

© The Author(s) 2025
B.-C. Liu (ed.), *Treatment of Refractory Renal Anemia*,
https://doi.org/10.1007/978-981-97-7636-8_32

reported infectious disease, trauma, blood transfusion, or known vaccination history. The patient had a penicillin allergy and denied any food allergies. She had no known exposure to epidemic or endemic sources, chemicals, dust, radiation, or toxic substances. She had no history of smoking, alcohol consumption, drug use, or travel. The patient's mother had hyperthyroidism, and her father had hypertension. Her vital signs included a temperature of 36.5 °C, pulse of 88 bpm, respiratory rate of 20 bpm, blood pressure of 160/88 mmHg, height of 155 cm, and weight of 55 kg. The patient appeared chronically ill with mild anemia, maintaining an autonomous position. Physical examination revealed no abnormalities in skin color, petechiae, ecchymosis, or palpable superficial lymph nodes. No facial edema or cyanosis of the lips was observed. Her neck was soft without resistance, and her thyroid gland was not enlarged. Auscultation revealed normal breath sounds, with no murmurs detected on cardiac auscultation. The abdomen was flat and soft with no tenderness or organomegaly. No deformities, redness, swelling, or tenderness of the joints was noted.

Her laboratory examinations showed the following results: WBC 8.51×10^9/L, RBC 3.63×10^{12}/L, Hb 115 g/L, platelets 126×10^9/L, neutrophil percentage 73.31%, creatinine 970.8 μmol/L, albumin 35.5 g/L, potassium 4.42 mmol/L, ALT 26 U/L, AST 22 U/L, glucose 5.33 mmol/L, $CO2$ 22.1 mmol/L, calcium 1.97 mmol/L, phosphorus 1.35 mmol/L, procalcitonin 1.07 ng/mL, ESR 50 mm/h, and CRP 8.46 mg/L. There were no abnormalities in tumor markers. Cardiac color Doppler ultrasound revealed aortic sclerosis, mild aortic valve degeneration, mild mitral and tricuspid insufficiency, and reduced left ventricular diastolic function. Chest and abdominal CT showed no significant abnormalities. Gastroscopy revealed chronic nonatrophic gastritis, while colonoscopy showed no significant findings.

She was given the following treatments: atorvastatin (20 mg, nightly), levamlodipine (2.5 mg, once daily), metoprolol sustained-release tablets (23.75 mg, once daily), perindopril tert-butylamine (8 mg, once daily) for hypertension, levothyroxine sodium (50 μg, once daily), calcitriol (5 μg, thrice weekly) for secondary hyperparathyroidism, and calcium acetate (0.6 g, once daily) for hyperphosphatemia.

32.1.1 Main Clinical Diagnosis

1. Chronic kidney disease stage 5 (maintenance hemodialysis).
2. Renal anemia and iron overload.
3. Renal hypertension.
4. Secondary hyperparathyroidism.
5. Hyperphosphatemia.
6. Hypothyroidism.

Atorvastatin (20 mg, once every night), levamlodipine (2.5 mg, once a day), metoprolol sustained-release tablets (23.75 mg, once a day), and perindopril tert-butylamine (8 mg, once a day) were used to treat hypertension. Levothyroxine sodium (50 μg, once a day) and calcitriol (5 μg, three times a week) were used to

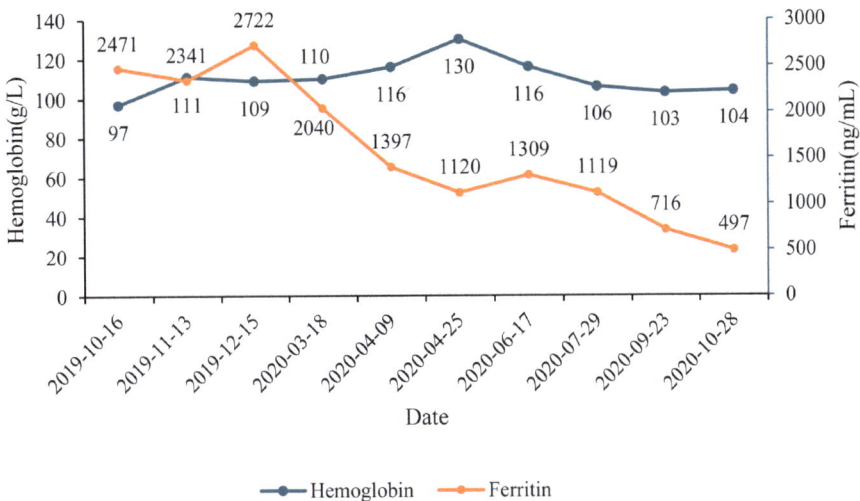

Fig. 32.1 Changes in hemoglobin and serum ferritin levels in patients from October 2019 to October 2020. Note: The patient was treated with rHuEPO from October 16, 2019 to March 17, 2020 and with roxadustat from March 18, 2020 to Oct 28, 2020

treat secondary hyperparathyroidism. Calcium acetate (0.6 g, once a day) was used to treat hyperphosphatemia.

32.1.2 Anemia Treatment

In December 2016, the patient's hemoglobin level was 92 g/L, and rHuEPO was administered at 4000 U thrice weekly. Later doses were adjusted based on her hemoglobin levels. In March 2020, the rHuEPO was discontinued, and roxadustat 100 mg was given thrice weekly. After gradual adjustment of the roxadustat dosage, her Hb level improved significantly, which was accompanied by a decrease in serum ferritin (Fig. 32.1).

32.2   Discussion

This elderly female patient on long-term maintenance hemodialysis presented with anemia and hyperferritinemia that were resistant to traditional ESA therapy. Roxadustat successfully increased her hemoglobin and decreased serum ferritin, suggesting its potential for treating ESA-resistant anemia by improving iron metabolism. The challenge in treating this patient was her body iron utilization disorder combined with hyperferritinemia, complicating the efficacy of ESA therapy. The success of roxadustat in this patient implies its utility in similar patients with ESA resistance, providing valuable clinical insights.

The challenge in treating this patient stems from an iron utilization disorder and hyperferritinemia, which contribute to the ineffectiveness of ESA therapy. Increasing functional iron without increasing the risk of iron accumulation is a major clinical consideration. The treatment of this patient demonstrated that roxadustat was able to increase the hemoglobin in an ESA-resistant patient by improving her iron metabolism.

Renal anemia is a common complication of CKD, its main causes being iron deficiency (absolute iron deficiency and functional iron deficiency), decreased erythropoiesis (EPO) production, ESA resistance, increased hepcidin, anemia due to inflammation, impaired hypoxia-inducible factor feedback loops, and vitamin D deficiency. Since its clinical application, rHuEPO and ESA have achieved good efficacy in the treatment of renal anemia, increasing hemoglobin levels, improving cardiovascular function, reducing blood transfusion rates, and delaying the progression of chronic kidney disease, but some patients still develop ESA hyporesponsiveness after long-term medication. Moreover, absolute or functional iron deficiency, vitamin deficiency, inflammatory response, malnutrition, inadequate dialysis, and secondary hyperparathyroidism (SHPT) are common causes of ESA hyporesponsiveness [1]. Patients on long-term maintenance hemodialysis are in a state of chronic microinflammation for a long time, which manifests as having many inflammatory markers in the blood, such as high-sensitivity C-reactive protein, IL-1, IL-6, IFN-γ, and TNF-α, which increase to varying degrees [2, 3].

Inflammation is closely associated with ESA hyporesponsiveness as well as functional iron deficiency. Hepcidin is produced by hepatocytes and can bind to surface membrane iron transporters located in duodenal epithelial cells, hepatocytes, and macrophages, inhibiting the absorption and utilization of intestinal iron and preventing iron from entering the blood circulation by promoting the internalization and degradation of membrane iron transporters [4]. When the body experiences inflammation or excess iron, hepcidin levels rise to lower blood iron, curb microbial growth, and prevent iron-related damage, while inflammation also causes iron retention in the reticuloendothelial system [5, 6]. In patients with CKD and end-stage renal disease, the glomerular filtration rate is decreased, and iron supplementation and inflammation can promote hepatic secretion of hepcidin [7]; therefore, CKD patients mostly have increased hepcidin levels. Roxadustat is an oral HIF-PHI that inhibits prolyl hydroxylase activity under normoxia to limit its degradation of HIF-1α, thereby stabilizing HIF-1α and letting it translocate to the nucleus to form stable functional heterodimers with HIF-1β to initiate the expression of genes downstream of HIF. Along with the genes encoding ESAs, these transcriptional targets include genes encoding divalent metal ion transporter (DMT1), duodenal cytochrome B (DcytB), transferrin, and transferrin receptor, which increase the body's absorption and transport of iron and improve iron metabolism in CKD patients. HIF promotes the release of erythropoietin from the bone marrow, which has a direct inhibitory effect on hepcidin. In addition, platelet-derived growth factor (PDGF)-BB inhibits hepcidin expression through the CREB/CREBH pathway [8]. Roxadustat can regulate erythropoiesis and correct anemia through multiple mechanisms; it improves hemoglobin without affecting the microinflammatory state. In a

26-week, randomized, multicenter, open-label, active-controlled, phase 3 study, roxadustat was able to reduce hepcidin levels in patients where epoetin alfa could not [9]. In this present case, long-term use of ESAs in maintenance hemodialysis patients was not effective, and the serum ferritin concentration continued to increase. After 6 months of roxadustat use, hemoglobin significantly improved, and serum ferritin significantly decreased. Later, the patient used ESA again due to external factors, and her iron utilization disorder and substandard hemoglobin recurred. These developments further confirmed that roxadustat can improve iron metabolism in the body and ameliorate anemia in ESA-resistant patients without influencing the body's inflammatory status.

The success of roxadustat in this patient suggests that it may increase hemoglobin in patients with ESA resistance by improving iron metabolism in the body, thus providing a reference for patients with similar conditions.

References

1. Alves MT, Vilaça SS, Carvalho M, Fernandes AP, Dusse LM, Gomes KB. Resistance of dialyzed patients to erythropoietin. Rev Bras Hematol Hemoter. 2015;37(3):190–7.
2. Johnson DW, Pascoe EM, Badve SV, et al. A randomized, placebo-controlled trial of pentoxifylline on erythropoiesis-stimulating agent hyporesponsiveness in anemic patients with CKD: the Handling Erythropoietin Resistance with Oxpentifylline (HERO) trial. Am J Kidney Dis. 2015;65(1):49–57.
3. Cooper AC, Mikhail A, Lethbridge MW, Kemeny DM, Macdougall IC. Increased expression of erythropoiesis inhibiting cytokines (IFN-gamma, TNF-alpha, IL-10, and IL-13) by T cells in patients exhibiting a poor response to erythropoietin therapy. J Am Soc Nephrol. 2003;14(7):1776–84.
4. El Sewefy DA, Farweez BA, Behairy MA, Yassin NR. Impact of serum hepcidin and inflammatory markers on resistance to erythropoiesis-stimulating therapy in haemodialysis patients. Int Urol Nephrol. 2019;51(2):325–34.
5. Gafter-Gvili A, Schechter A, Rozen-Zvi B. Iron deficiency Anemia in chronic kidney disease. Acta Haematol. 2019;142(1):44–50.
6. Małyszko J, Koc-Żórawska E, Levin-Iaina N, et al. New parameters in iron metabolism and functional iron deficiency in patients on maintenance hemodialysis. Pol Arch Med Wewn. 2012;122(11):537–42.
7. Rytkönen KT, Williams TA, Renshaw GM, Primmer CR, Nikinmaa M. Molecular evolution of the metazoan PHD-HIF oxygen-sensing system. Mol Biol Evol. 2011;28(6):1913–26.
8. Pasricha SR, McHugh K, Drakesmith H. Regulation of hepcidin by erythropoiesis: the story so far. Annu Rev Nutr. 2016;36:417–34.
9. Chen N, Hao C, Liu BC, et al. Roxadustat treatment for anemia in patients undergoing long-term dialysis. N Engl J Med. 2019;381(11):1011–22.

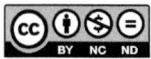

Conventional Dose of Roxadustat Causes Hyperhemoglobinemia in a Peritoneal Dialysis Patient with Renal Anemia

33

Qing Yin, Bi-Cheng Liu, and Bin Wang

33.1 Case Presentation

A 58-year-old man presented to our hospital because of foamy urine for 10 years, poor food intake, and fatigue for 2 years. The patient was diagnosed with diabetic nephropathy 10 years ago due to proteinuria. Two years before admission, the patient's symptoms worsened with serum creatinine elevation, and he developed symptoms of poor food intake and fatigue, and the diagnosis of "chronic kidney disease (CKD) stage 5 and diabetic kidney disease (V)" was made. He was initially treated with peritoneal dialysis. The patient's ambulatory peritoneal dialysis regimen was a low-calcium peritoneal dialysate (lactate −1.5%), 2 L of which was retained in the abdominal cavity for 4 hours at a time. His daily peritoneal dialysis ultrafiltration volume was 400 mL to 700 mL. His daily urine output is about 300 mL to 500 mL.

The patient had a 10-year history of diabetes, which was treated with subcutaneous administration of recombinant insulin. He also had an 8-year history of hypertension, for which he regularly took antihypertensive drugs (sacubitril valsartan sodium tablets). He had a history of "coronary heart disease and percutaneous coronary intervention" for 3 years and was treated with aspirin and statins orally. His blood pressure was 151/84 mmHg, and his body weight was 55 kg. Physical examination showed systemic pigmentation, regular heart rhythm, and no rales on both sides of the chest. There was no edema in both lower limbs.

Q. Yin · B.-C. Liu (✉) · B. Wang
Institute of Nephrology, Zhong Da Hospital, Southeast University School of Medicine, Nanjing, China

© The Author(s) 2025
B.-C. Liu (ed.), *Treatment of Refractory Renal Anemia*,
https://doi.org/10.1007/978-981-97-7636-8_33

203

Laboratory examinations at admission revealed the following: white blood cell (WBC) count, 5.11×10^9/L; red blood cell (RBC) count, 6.95×10^{12}/L; hemoglobin, 212 g/L; platelet count, 68×10^9/L; erythropoietin (EPO), 147.50 mIU/mL↑; C-reactive protein, 1.42 mg/L; serum total protein, 45.8 g/L; albumin, 22.4 g/L; blood urea nitrogen, 20.7 mmol/L; creatinine, 695 μmol/L (reference range, 57–111 μmol/L); serum potassium, 3.01 mmol/L; calcium, 1.87 mmol/L; phosphorus, 2.73 mmol/L; uric acid, 181 μmol/L; parathyroid hormone, 329.47 pg/mL; β2 microglobulin, 45.0 mg/L; D-dimer, 1838 μg/L; TnI, 0.036 ng/mL; MYO, >900 ng/mL; and CKMB, 100 ng/mL. No abnormalities of vascular embolism, tumor mass, and splenomegaly were found in imaging examination.

In addition, biomarkers of iron status, including stored iron and functional iron, were measured (iron, 20.1 μmol/L; transferrin saturation, 49.0%; total iron-binding capacity, 39.4 μmol/L; and ferritin, 61.74 μg/L). To explore the cause of anemia, bone marrow puncture was performed. The patient's bone marrow showed that granuloid and erythroid were not significantly abnormal, but the megakaryocyte maturation was impaired (platelets scattered).

We reviewed the hemoglobin changes of the patients in the past 2 years (Fig. 33.1). At the beginning, his hemoglobin was 85 g/L when he entered peritoneal dialysis, and it steadily increased to 132 g/L after oral administration of roxadustat. During the administration of roxadustat, its dosage was incrementally regulated in accordance with the patient's hemoglobin levels. Regrettably, the patient exhibited poor compliance, failing to attend the clinic on a regular basis for necessary follow-ups and consequent dosage adjustments. This lapse led to the development of hyperhemoglobinemia, with the patient's hemoglobin reaching as high as 195–212 g/L. Fortunately, after stopping the use of roxadustat, his hemoglobin level gradually decreased, and he showed no other side effects such as thromboembolism.

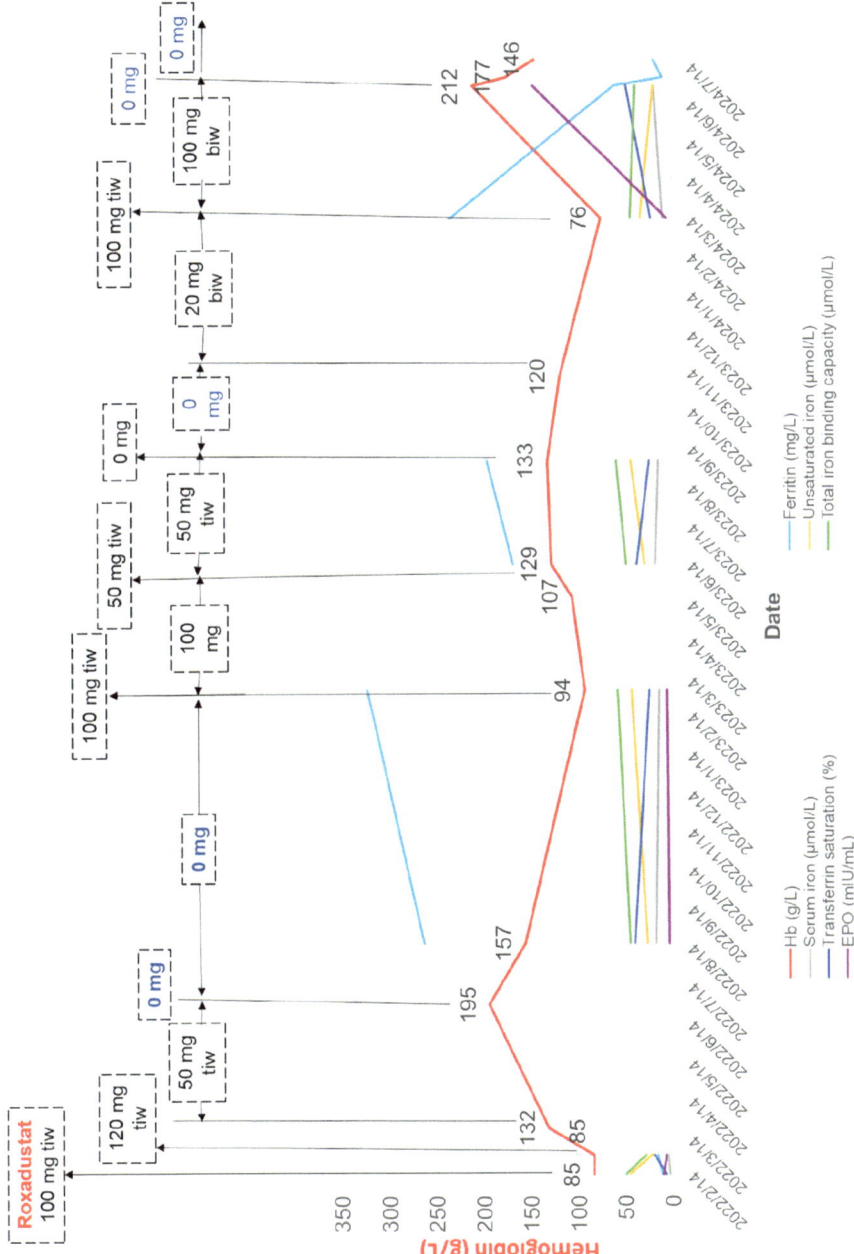

Fig. 33.1 Adjustment process of roxadustat administration and changes in hemoglobin levels and iron metabolism

33.2 Discussion

This case involves a middle-aged male patient on peritoneal dialysis who presented with moderate to severe anemia and a history of type 2 diabetes and hypertension. The patient responded well to the treatment of roxadustat, with a gradual increase in hemoglobin to 120 g/L to 130 g/L. Unfortunately, due to the patient's failure to regularly visit the outpatient clinic for blood routine testing and timely adjustment of the dose, he presented with extremely high hemoglobin level.

Renal anemia is a common and important complication in patients with CKD, which not only affects the patient's quality of life, but also promotes the progression of kidney disease and increases the risk of cardiovascular events and death [1, 2]. The incidence of renal anemia is high in China, but the rate of treatment is low. The etiology of CKD anemia is multifactorial, including EPO deficiency, abnormal iron metabolism, chronic inflammation, and blood loss, among which EPO deficiency is the most specific [3, 4]. In the past 30 years, the use of erythropoiesis-stimulating agent (ESA) and iron has significantly improved the prognosis of CKD patients, but some patients still have low ESA response or multiple adverse reactions due to various reasons, and new treatment strategies are urgently needed [5].

Roxadustat is the first approved hypoxia-inducing factor prolyl hydroxylase inhibitor (HIF-PHI) [6, 7]. It can stabilize the expression of HIF by inhibiting the activity of PHD, so that HIF can directly and specifically bind the HIF-binding site of EPO gene in the kidney and liver and promote the expression of EPO. Moreover, roxadustat promotes the release of iron from hepatocytes and macrophages by downregulating hepcidin, increasing the availability of iron in the body, and ultimately improving iron metabolism disorders [8]. Therefore, roxadustat improves renal anemia by mimicking the natural response to hypoxia and improving iron metabolism.

Our case report shows that routinely recommended dose of roxadustat causes hyperhemoglobinemia in peritoneal dialysis patients with renal anemia. After discontinuation of the drug, the patient's hyperhemoglobinemia returned to the normal within 2 months. Despite the occurrence of hyperhemoglobinemia, we observed a surprising effect of roxadustat on improving iron metabolism (Fig. 33.1).

During the treatment, 100 mg of roxadustat was used three times a week, and after 3 months, the patient showed a significant increase in iron utilization, manifested by a significant reduction in ferritin (236.16 mg/L to 61.74 mg/L) and a significant increase in transferrin saturation (22.9% to 49%). In addition, roxadustat significantly increased EPO levels in this patient (6.43 mIU/mL to 147.5 mIU/mL) and ultimately significantly increased hemoglobin. The patient was prescribed the regular dosage of roxadustat. However, it led to a remarkably high hemoglobin level, while fortunately, no cardiovascular diseases like vascular embolism occurred. This case underlines the significance of regularly tracking the changes in the patient's hemoglobin level and making personalized adjustments to the roxadustat dosage to guarantee both the safety and efficacy of the treatment.

In summary, our study revealed that roxadustat could effectively improve the anemia status of peritoneal dialysis patients. Roxadustat significantly reduces ferritin and keeps transferrin saturation stable, allowing more iron stored in the body to participate in hematopoiesis. It can also reduce the use of exogenous iron agents and lessen the risk of iron overload, thereby improving the utilization rate of iron. Therefore, roxadustat could be an ideal alterative therapy for renal anemia. The particular implication for this case is that the dosage of roxadustat should be individualized by carefully monitoring the hemoglobin level, because some patient may respond to the therapy quickly and potentially cause hyperhemoglobinemia.

References

1. Chen N, Hao C, Liu BC, et al. Roxadustat treatment for anemia in patients undergoing long-term dialysis. N Engl J Med. 2019;381:1011–22.
2. Chen N, Hao C, Peng X, et al. Roxadustat for anemia in patients with kidney disease not receiving dialysis. N Engl J Med. 2019;381:1001–10.
3. Jodie LB, Herbert YL. Mechanisms of anemia in CKD. J Am Soc Nephrol. 2012;23:1631–4.
4. Bazeley JW, Wish JB. Recent and emerging therapies for iron deficiency in anemia of CKD: a review. Am J Kidney Dis. 2022;79:868–76.
5. Wu H, Chinnadurai R. Erythropoietin-stimulating agent hyporesponsiveness in patients living with chronic kidney disease. Kidney Dis (Basel). 2022;8:103–14.
6. Gupta N, Wish JB. Hypoxia-inducible factor prolyl hydroxylase inhibitors: a potential new treatment for anemia in patients with CKD. Am J Kidney Dis. 2017;69:815–26.
7. Haase VH. Hypoxia-inducible factor-prolyl hydroxylase inhibitors in the treatment of anemia of chronic kidney disease. Kidney Int Suppl (2011). 2021;11:8–25.
8. Sanghani NS, Haase VH. Hypoxia-inducible factor activators in renal anemia: current clinical experience. Adv Chronic Kidney Dis. 2019;26:253–66.

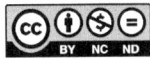